POCKET GUIDE
TO BREAST CANCER

Second Edition

Jones and Bartlett Series in Oncology

POCKET GUIDE TO BREAST CANCER

Second Edition

Edited by

KAREN HASSEY DOW, PhD, RN, FAAN

Associate Professor
School of Nursing, College of Health and Public Affairs
University of Central Florida
Orlando, Florida

JONES AND BARTLETT PUBLISHERS
Sudbury, Massachusetts
Boston   Toronto   London   Singapore

World Headquarters

Jones and Bartlett Publishers
40 Tall Pine Drive
Sudbury, MA 01776
978-443-5000
www.jbpub.com
info@jbpub.com

Jones and Bartlett Publishers Canada
2406 Nikanna Road
Mississauga, ON L5C 2W6
CANADA

Jones and Bartlett Publishers International
Barb House, Barb Mews
London W6 7PA
UK

Production Credits

Acquisitions Editor: Penny Glynn
Associate Editor: Thomas Prindle
Production Editor: Jon Workman
Marketing Manager: Taryn Wahlquist
V.P., Manufacturing Buyer and Inventory Control: Therese Bräuer
Editorial and Production Service: Colophon
Composition: Modern Graphics
Printing and Binding: United Graphics
Cover Design: Philip Regan

Library of Congress Cataloging-in-Publication Data

Dow, Karen Hassey.
    Pocket guide to breast cancer / by Karen Hassey Dow.—2nd ed.
        p. ; cm.
    Includes bibliographical references and index.
    ISBN 0-7637-1814-9 (pbk.)
        1. Breast—Cancer—Nursing—Handbooks, manuals, etc.
    I. Contemporary issues in breast cancer.   II. Title.
        [DNLM: 1. Breast Neoplasms—nursing—Handbooks. WP 39 D744p
    2002]
    RC280.B8 D67 2002
    616.99'449—dc21   2002041284

Printed in the United States of America
05 04 03 02 01   10 9 8 7 6 5 4 3 2 1

With love and appreciation for my mother Nena and in loving memory of my father Orlando.

Contents

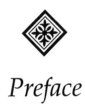

Preface

Welcome to the second edition of the *Pocket Guide*. This edition is similar to the first edition, with the goal of providing an easy-to-use, day-to-day reference for nurses caring for patients with breast cancer and their families. Similar to the first edition, the content of the *Pocket Guide* is divided into four parts: Epidemiology, Screening, Early Detection and Diagnosis; Treatment of Primary Breast Cancer; Treatment of Recurrent and Metastatic Breast Cancer; and Quality-of-Life Issues. The chapters have been updated to provide the reader with current information. The reader should keep in mind that breast cancer care is undergoing rapid developments and changes. Individual, programmatic, and institutional differences in the care of patients with breast cancer may vary.

Acknowledgments

Thanks to Penny Glynn and Christine Tridente for their patience and encouragement in this project. And heart-felt thanks to my husband Norman and daughter Lauren for their love and support.

Disclaimer

Given the tremendous breakthroughs in cancer research and changes in clinical practice, the nature of breast cancer care is constantly evolving. The information about drug dosages presented in this pocket guide is in accord with recommendations at the time of publication. The editor and publisher have made every effort to provide accurate information. However, before administering any drug, the reader is advised to check the manufacturer's product information sheet for the most current recommendations on dosage, precautions, and contraindications. The reader is advised that the authors, editor, reviewers, and publisher cannot be responsible for any errors or omissions in this handbook, or for any consequences arising therefrom.

PART I

Epidemiology, Screening, Early Detection, and Diagnosis

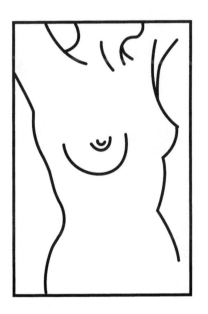

1

Incidence, Epidemiology, and Survival

❖ Trends in Incidence

- ✦ Most common cancer in American women[1]
- ✦ 193,700 estimated new cases for 2001

  192,200 new cases in women

  1,500 new cases in men

- ✦ Accounts for 31% of new cancer cases in American women in 2001

- ✦ Incidence rates of invasive breast cancer in the United States were the same during the 1990s.

  Incidence is decreasing in younger women.

- ✦ Overall case rate per 100,000 age-adjusted women was 118.4 for Whites and 103.0 for Blacks.

- ✦ Worldwide, incidence increased 0.5% annually, with 1.35 to 1.45 million new cases projected by 2010.

❖ **Survival**

✦ Five-year relative survival rate for all women with localized invasive breast cancer is 96.5%, based on the National Cancer Institute's Surveillance, Epidemiology, and End Results (SEER) program.[2]

✦ Five-year survival rate for all stages is 85%.

✦ Survival decreases with advanced stage of disease at diagnosis.

❖ **Mortality**

✦ Estimated 40,600 deaths due to breast cancer in 2001

40,200 deaths in women

400 deaths in men

✦ Second leading cause of cancer deaths in American women after lung cancer

✦ Leading cause of cancer death in women age 40 to 59

✦ Accounts for 15% of all cancer deaths in American women

✦ Breast cancer deaths have declined.

1995 deaths due to breast cancer were 43,844.

1998 deaths due to breast cancer were 41,737.

✦ Factors relating to decreased mortality

Mammographic screening[3]

TABLE 1-1
Ten-Year Survival by Stage[4]

Stage	10-Year Survival
0	95%
I	88%
II	66%
III	36%
IV	7%

> *Systemic therapy*
>
> *Improved understanding of the mechanisms of recurrence and metastasis*

+ Highest decrease in mortality occurred in White women and younger women.

+ Table 1-1 shows ten-year survival by stage.

+ Worldwide, 1% to 2% reduction in mortality in countries having a high incidence, such as the United States, Canada, and the United Kingdom[5]

+ Japan, Italy, Spain, Portugal, Greece, Hungary, and Poland have an increase in mortality.

+ No change in mortality in non-developed countries in Asia, Latin America, and Africa.

❖ **Racial and Ethnic Differences**

+ Incidence and mortality rates vary by race and ethnicity.

+ White women have a higher incidence than women of any other racial or ethnic group.[6]

+ Black women have a higher mortality from breast cancer, compared with any other racial or ethnic group.

+ Black women have a poorer probability of survival once they are diagnosed.

+ Factors associated with higher mortality in Black women

  Later stage at diagnosis

  Disease characteristics such as larger tumor size, greater nodal involvement, estrogen receptor (ER)–negative tumors, shorter time to recurrence

  Limited access to breast cancer screening, less than adequate treatment, and social and economic factors

TABLE 1-2
Incidence and Mortality Rates by Race and Ethnicity, United States: 1990–1997[1]

Racial/Ethnic Group	Incidence	Mortality
White	114.0	25.3
Black	100.2	31.4
Asian/Pacific Islander	74.6	11.2
Native American	33.4	12.1
Hispanic	68.9	15.1

◆ Table 1-2 shows the incidence and mortality by ethnic group.

REFERENCES

1. Greenlee, R., Hill-Harmon, M., Murray, T., & Thun, M. (2001). Cancer statistics, 2001. *CA: A Cancer Journal for Clinicians, 51*, 15–37.

2. SEER online at http://www-seer.ims.nci.nih.gov/

3. Del Turco, M. R. (1999). Breast cancer update: Encouraging trends—many new questions. *CA: A Cancer Journal for Clinicians, 49*, 135–137.

4. Fremgen, A., Bland, K., McGinnis, L., Jr., et al. (1999). Clinical highlights from the National Cancer Data Base, 1999. *CA: A Cancer Journal for Clinicians, 49*, 145–158.

5. Mettlin, C. (1999). Global breast cancer mortality statistics. *CA: A Cancer Journal for Clinicians, 49*, 138–144.

6. Dignam, J. J. (2000). Differences in breast cancer prognosis among African-American and Caucasian women. *CA: A Cancer Journal for Clinicians, 50*, 50–64.

2

Nongenetic and Heritable Risk Factors

❖ Background

- ✦ Risk factors, both nongenetic and inherited, pose a major concern and source of confusion among women.

- ✦ Individual rather than epidemiologic risk factors are discussed in this chapter.

- ✦ About 90% of all breast cancers are sporadic, with about 10% inherited.

❖ Major Risk Factors

- ✦ Female gender

    Of the 193,700 estimated new cases for 2001, 192,200 new cases are projected in women, with only 1,500 new cases projected in men.

    Breast cancer is rare among men.

✦ Advancing age

> *Breast cancer is rare among women younger than age 20 years.*
>
> *Incidence increases with age, with a large increase by age 50.*
>
> *Risk is 1 in 39 before age 50.*
>
> *Risk is 1 in 29 before age 60.*
>
> *Risk is 1 in 8 by age 86.*

✦ Family history of breast cancer

> *Increased risk when breast cancer occurs in first-degree relative (i.e., mother, sister, or daughter)*

✦ Benign proliferative disease

> *Atypical hyperplasia*
>
> 1. Women with atypical hyperplasia are four to five times more likely to develop breast cancer.
>
> 2. Risk may decrease after menopause.
>
> *Lobular carcinoma in situ (LCIS)*
>
> 1. Considered a marker or risk factor rather than a precursor to breast cancer
>
> 2. Women with LCIS have an increased risk of 1% per year for developing breast cancer.
>
> 3. Lesion is usually asymptomatic,

incidental microscopic finding that does not show as a mass on mammography.

4. Seen more often in younger than older women

❖ **Reproductive Risk Factors**[1]

+ Age at menarche

    Early menarche at ages 11 to 15 increases risk.

    Shorter menstrual cycles are associated with increase in breast cancer risk.

    Long and irregular cycles are associated with reduced breast cancer risk.

    Early menarche and late menopause are related to increased total lifetime number of menstrual cycles, with a corresponding 30% to 50% increase in breast cancer risk.

    Long exposure to estrogen with uninterrupted menstrual cycles is thought to be a mechanism for increased risk.

+ Nulliparity is an increased risk, compared with parity, and this risk is evident after 40 to 45 years of age.

+ First full-term pregnancy after age 30

+ Age at menopause

    Late menopause after age 55 increases risk.

    Women having bilateral oophorectomy before age 45

have one-half the risk of breast cancer, compared with women having natural menopause at age 55 years or older.

Risk of breast cancer increases by about 3% per year when age at menopause is delayed.

Reduction in risk with early menopause is likely a result of the cessation of breast cell division and the decline in endogenous hormone levels.

+ Prenatal exposure to estrogen

   Strong inverse relationship seen between presence of preeclampsia and decreased risk of breast cancer

+ Induced abortion

   Conflicting evidence regarding increased risk after therapeutic abortion, although the available evidence does not demonstrate a relationship between induced abortion and risk

❖ Exogenous Hormone Risk Factors

+ Several meta-analyses of women who had ever used oral contraceptives did not show an association with breast cancer risk.

+ The drawback of these studies showed a range of "ever use" from short-term to long-term use.

   There is an increased risk among young women who use oral contraceptives for a long period of time.

+ Studies indicate that there is no increased risk of

breast cancer in women using hormone replacement therapy (HRT), compared with women who have never used HRT.

> *An increased risk is observed in users of long duration and current users.*

❖ Energy Expenditure as Risk Factors

+ Weight gain

    > *High-energy intake that accelerates growth and earlier menstruation in childhood and weight gain in middle life increase the risk of breast cancer.*

+ Decreased or lack of physical activity may have a relationship to weight gain and increased risk of postmenopausal breast cancer.

❖ Dietary Risk Factors

+ High intake of dietary fat does not increase risk of breast cancer.

+ Alcohol intake of more than two drinks per day increases risk.

    > *Moderate alcohol intake increases endogenous estrogen levels and shows the clearest relationship between diet and breast cancer risk.*

+ Dietary fiber; micronutrients, including vitamins A, E, and C; and selenium do not support a protective factor from breast cancer.

+ Caffeine intake through drinking coffee or tea does not demonstrate an increased risk of breast cancer.

❖ **Environmental Risk Factors**

+ Radiation therapy at a young age

   Young women exposed to ionizing radiation to the chest at a young age for treatment of Hodgkin's disease have an excess risk of breast cancer.

+ Electromagnetic field exposure does not indicate a link to increased breast cancer risk.

+ Environmental exposure to pesticides and organochlorines does not appear to be a major risk factor in development of breast cancer.

❖ **A Model for Risk Assessment**

+ Gail Risk Assessment Model is a statistical model to assess a woman's individualized absolute risk (i.e., chance that a woman with specific risk factors at a given age will develop breast cancer in a specific future time period).

+ Women are considered at high risk for breast cancer when their risk is equal to or greater than that of the average 60-year-old woman.

+ Factors used in determining risk

   Current age

   Race

   Age at menarche

Age at first live birth (or nulliparity)

Number of breast biopsies

Atypical hyperplasia

Number of first-degree relatives with breast cancer (i.e., mother, sister, daughters)

+ Model has been validated in women undergoing regular mammography screening.

+ Risk assessment available for White, non-Black women, and Black women

+ Gail Risk Assessment Model available from the National Cancer Institute website: http://www.nci.nih.gov

❖ **Inherited Risk Factors[2]**

+ Breast cancer susceptibility genes are responsible for 5% to 10% of all breast cancers.

+ There are two types of genetic damage responsible for the development of the malignant phenotype:

Activation of proto-oncogenes

Inactivation of tumor-suppressor genes

Mutated tumor-suppressor genes lose critical functions in regulating the cell cycle, cellular response to DNA damage, and preventing the mutation of other critical genes.

+ Presence of gene mutation BRCA1 or BRCA2

Inherited gene mutation occurs in 1 in 200 women.

Inherited gene mutation occurs in 1 in 40 women of Eastern European descent.

Gene mutation inherited from either parent

BRCA1 mutation increases chance of breast cancer by 35% to 85%. BRCA2 mutation increases chance of breast cancer by 20% to 60%.

❖ BRCA1

- ✦ BRCA1 is located on chromosome 17q21, and this mutation is associated with early-onset breast cancer.

- ✦ BRCA1 is associated with an increased risk of ovarian cancer.

- ✦ BRCA1 tumors tend to have aggressive pathologic features, such as high nuclear-grade, and are often estrogen-receptor negative and progesterone-receptor negative.

❖ BRCA2

- ✦ Mutations may contribute to fewer cases of early-onset breast cancer, compared with BRCA1.

- ✦ BRCA2 mutations are associated with an elevated risk for the development of other cancers, such as prostate, pancreatic, non-Hodgkin's lymphoma, and bladder cancer.

+ BRCA2 mutations are associated with a 6% lifetime risk of male breast cancer.

❖ **Other Inherited Genetic Factors[3]**

+ Li-Fraumeni syndrome

> *Autosomal dominant disorder associated with increased risk of several tumors, including soft-tissue sarcomas, breast cancer, osteosarcoma, adrenocortical carcinoma, brain tumors, acute leukemia, and possibly other cancers*

> *Fifty percent of patients have germline mutations that fall within a single small region on the p53 tumor-suppressor gene.*

> *About 50% of women with the Li-Fraumeni syndrome may develop breast cancer. This disorder probably affects less than 1% of all breast cancer cases.*

+ Ataxia-telangiectasia

> *Autosomal recessive disorder characterized by the development of cerebellar ataxia, telangiectases, immune defects, and predisposition to malignancy.*

> *Affected individuals have a 10% to 20% risk of developing cancer, especially lymphomas and lymphocytic leukemias, but also epithelial tumors, including breast cancer.*

Relatives of individuals with ataxia-telangiectasia appear to have an increased risk of breast cancer.

+ Muir-Torre syndrome

    Rare autosomal dominant condition that includes multiple benign sebaceous adenomas and carcinomas, basal and squamous cell carcinomas, and keratoacanthomas of the skin, as well as multiple internal malignancies

    Inherited cancers include tumors of the colon, stomach, esophagus, breast, uterus, ovaries, bladder, and larynx, as well as squamous cell carcinoma of the mucous membranes.

+ Cowden's syndrome

    Autosomal dominant trait is characterized by multiple hamartomatous lesions of skin, mucous membranes, breast, and thyroid.

    Fifty percent of affected females have fibrocystic disease of the breast as well as breast cancer, of which 33% are bilateral breast cancer.

    Increased incidence of cancers of the thyroid, colon, uterus, cervix, lung, bladder, skin, and lymphoreticular system

+ Peutz-Jeghers syndrome

    Autosomal dominant disorder is characterized by the association of black or bluish melanin spots on the lips, perioral region, buccal mucosa, hands, arms, feet, and legs, with gastrointestinal polyposis.

Syndrome carries increased risk of cancers of the breast, uterus, and ovarian sex cord.

❖ Risk Counseling and Predisposition Testing[4,5]

✦ Risk counseling

Evaluation of family history in at least two generations

Predisposition testing is helpful when family member with breast cancer undergoes the initial testing.

Age, education, and previous diagnosis of cancer are important aspects in decision-making after positive genetic testing.

Elements of informed consent must be considered for an individual considering testing for cancer susceptibility.

1. Information about the tests, risks, benefits, and efficacy

2. Option of risk estimation without genetic testing

3. Risk of passing a mutation to the next generation

4. Technical accuracy (sensitivity and specificity) of testing

5. Options for risk management, including increased surveillance and screening

6. Psychosocial risks and distress

7. Potential for work-related discrimination

8. Costs of testing and counseling

Breast cancer risk assessment is ideally done by using a multidisciplinary approach.

✦ Management

Close surveillance, education, and counseling

Prophylactic mastectomy may be considered as an option.

REFERENCES

1. Willett, W., Rockhill, B., Hankinson, S., et al. (2000). Epidemiology and nongenetic causes of breast cancer. In J. R. Harris, M. Lippman, M. Morrow, & C. K. Osborne (Eds.), *Diseases of the breast* (2nd ed., pp. 175–220). Philadelphia: Lippincott Williams & Wilkins.

2. DeMichele, A., & Weber, B. (2000). Inherited genetic factors. In J. R. Harris, M. Lippman, M. Morrow, & C. K. Osborne (Eds.), *Diseases of the breast* (2nd ed., pp. 221–236). Philadelphia: Lippincott Williams & Wilkins.

3. Strauss-Trainin, A. (1996). Genetics and breast cancer risk. In K. H. Dow (Ed.), *Contemporary issues in breast cancer* (pp. 3–19). Sudbury, MA: Jones and Bartlett.

4. Metcalfe, K., Liede, A., Hoodfar, E., et al. (2000). An evaluation of needs of female BRCA1 and BRCA2 carriers undergoing genetic counseling. *Journal of Medical Genetics, 37*, 866–874.

5. Cummings, S., & Olopade, O. (1998). Predisposition testing for inherited breast cancer. *Oncology, 12,* 1227–1242.

3

Prevention Strategies

- ✦ There is no one specific, proven method of preventing breast cancer.[1]

- ✦ All women can limit their risk factors in a variety of ways.

- ✦ Women at high risk may be candidates for chemoprevention or risk-reducing surgery.

- ✦ All women can practice lifestyle modification.

❖ Approaches to Prevention

- ✦ Chemoprevention

- ✦ Risk-reducing surgery

- ✦ Lifestyle modification

❖ Chemoprevention

- ✦ Definition: Use of a drug to reduce cancer risk

  Example: Tamoxifen, which is an estrogen antagonist and agonist

✦ Breast Cancer Prevention Trial P-1 (BCPT)[2]

> *Over 13,000 women at increased risk (i.e., at least 60 years of age or 35–59 years with predicted risk of at least 1.66 on Gail Model) randomized to receive either tamoxifen 20 mg daily or placebo for 5 years*

> *Risk of invasive breast cancer reduced by 49% in women receiving tamoxifen*

> *Women with atypical hyperplasia had an 86% reduction in risk.*

> *Tamoxifen did not affect the incidence of estrogen receptor (ER)–negative tumors.*

> *Women with lobular carcinoma in situ (LCIS) had a 56% reduction in risk.*

> *Increased risk of endometrial cancer,[3] deep vein thrombosis (DVT), and pulmonary embolism of less than 1% while on tamoxifen*

> *Beneficial effects of tamoxifen included a reduction in hip, radius, and spine fractures.*

> *Conclusion that tamoxifen decreased the incidence of invasive and non-invasive breast cancer and is an appropriate preventive agent in women at increased risk*

> *Tamoxifen is approved in the United States for reduction of breast cancer risk in women at high risk.*

> *Tamoxifen therapy lasts for 5 years, and, thus, risk reduction must be weighed against potential risks of long-term drug usage.*[4]

✦ Study of raloxifene and tamoxifen (STAR)

> *Multiple Outcomes of Raloxifene Evaluation (MORE) was a trial designed to evaluate the effect of raloxifene in preventing bone fractures in post-menopausal women treated with 60 or 120 mg/day, the relative risk of breast cancer was 0.24 in the raloxifene group.*[5]

> *STAR is a randomized, double-blind clinical trial of 22,000 women.*

> *Purpose is to compare raloxifene and tamoxifen as chemopreventive agents in high-risk women.*

> *First trial to incorporate an active agent (tamoxifen instead of placebo) as the standard of care*

> *To date, approximately 1.7% of women are African-American; 1.3% are Hispanic/Latina; and 1.6% are of other ethnic minority heritage.*

> *Information about STAR trial is available at the National Surgical Adjuvant Breast and Bowel Project website (http://www.nsabp.pitt.edu).*

❖ **Risk-Reducing Surgery**

✦ Bilateral prophylactic mastectomy reduces breast cancer risk.

+ However, no mastectomy can remove all existing mammary tissue.

+ Prophylactic mastectomy is associated with a 90% reduction in the incidence of breast cancer.[6]

+ Drawbacks relate to disfigurement and potential psychological trauma.

+ Candidates for bilateral prophylactic mastectomy

  Strong family or personal history of breast cancer

  Multiple previous breast biopsies

  Diagnosis of LCIS or atypical hyperplasia

  Inherited susceptibility

+ Nurse's role in risk-reducing surgery[7]

  Facilitate referral to plastic surgeon to evaluate reconstructive options.

  Explore potential psychological and social effects of prophylactic and bilateral mastectomy.

  Educate the patient about the surgical procedure and potential complications, including bleeding, infection, and flap reconstruction loss.

❖ **Lifestyle Modification**

+ No lifestyle modification has yet been shown to prevent breast cancer.

+ Breast cancer risk may be reduced by lifestyle modification such as

> *Weight control and reduction*
>
> *Smoking cessation*
>
> *Decreased alcohol consumption*
>
> *Exercise*

❖ Weight Control

- ✦ Obesity is associated with an increased risk of breast cancer in post-menopausal women.

- ✦ Fat stores provide an important source of hormone substrates in post-menopausal women.

- ✦ Reducing body weight may potentially lower breast cancer risk. The American Cancer Society recommends that women maintain a healthy weight and limit intake of high-fat, animal sources of food.

- ✦ Areas of interest identified by women include changes in dietary fat consumption, use of calcium supplements and natural and herbal remedies, and evaluation of soy products and phytoestrogens in the diet.

❖ Smoking Cessation

- ✦ Smoking increases risk of lung and other cancers and increases risk of heart disease.

- ✦ Smoking affects overall health but has not had a direct effect on the development of breast cancer.

❖ **Alcohol Consumption**

✦ Moderate to high amounts of alcohol consumption have been associated with increased breast cancer incidence.[8]

✦ Mechanisms by which ethanol may increase risk[1]

Induces increased levels of circulating estrogen

Stimulates hepatic metabolism of carcinogens

Facilitates transport of carcinogens into breast tissue

Modulates cell membrane integrity with an effect on carcinogenesis

Aids production of cytotoxic protein products

Impairs immune surveillance

Promotes production of toxic congeners

Increases exposure to toxic oxidants

Reduces intake and bioavailability of protective nutrients

❖ **Exercise**

✦ Exercise may reduce the risk of breast cancer and is associated with enhanced immune function, lower body fat, and hormonal levels.

✦ Decreased risk of breast cancer is associated with increasing amounts of physical activity.[9]

✦ Greater leisure-time activity is associated with 37% reduction in relative risk of breast cancer for women who regularly exercised, compared with sedentary women, with risk reduction greatest in premenopausal women.[10]

REFERENCES

1. Vogel, V. (2000). Breast cancer prevention: A review of current evidence. *CA: A Cancer Journal for Clinicians, 50,* 156–170.

2. Fisher, B., Costantino, J., Wickerham, D., et al. (1998). Tamoxifen for prevention of breast cancer: Report of the National Surgical Adjuvant Breast and Bowel Project P-1 Study. *Journal of the National Cancer Institute, 16,* 1381–1388.

3. Fisher, B., Costantino, J., Redmond, C., et al. (1994). Endometrial cancer in tamoxifen-treated breast cancer patients: Findings from the National Surgical Adjuvant Breast and Bowel Project (NSABP) B-14. *Journal of the National Cancer Institute, 86,* 527–537.

4. Gail, M., Costantino, J., Bryant, J., et al. (1999). Weighing the risks and benefits of tamoxifen treatment for preventing breast cancer. *Journal of the National Cancer Institute, 91,* 1829–1846.

5. Cummings, S., Eckert, S., Krueger, K., et al. (1999). The effect of raloxifene on risk of breast cancer in post-menopausal women: Results from the MORE randomized trial. Multiple Outcomes of Raloxifene Evaluation. *Journal of the American Medical Association, 281,* 2189–2197.

6. Hartmann, L., Schaid, D., & Woods, J. (1999). Efficacy of bilateral prophylactic mastectomy in women with a family history of breast cancer. *New England Journal of Medicine, 340*, 77–84.

7. Gross, R. (2000). Breast cancer: Risk factors, screening, and prevention. *Seminars in Oncology Nursing, 16*, 176–184.

8. Smith-Warner, S., Spiegelman, D., Yaunn, S., et al. (1998). Alcohol and breast cancer in women: A pooled analysis of cohort studies. *Journal of the American Medical Association, 279*, 535–540.

9. Bernstein, L., Henderson, B., Hanisch, R., et al. (1994). Physical exercise and reduced risk of breast cancer in young women. *Journal of the National Cancer Institute, 86*, 1403–1408.

10. Thune, I., Brenn, T., Lund, E., et al. (1997). Physical activity and the risk of breast cancer. *New England Journal of Medicine, 336*, 1269–1275.

4

Screening and Early Detection

❖ **Principles of Cancer Screening**[1]

- ✦ Distinguish among individuals who are likely and not likely to have the disease.

- ✦ Criteria for screening

    Disease must be an important health problem.

    Disease must be the period when the disease is detectable in an asymptomatic individual.

    Screening test must be effective, accurate, and affordable.

❖ **Goals of Breast Cancer Screening**

- ✦ Earlier diagnosis in asymptomatic individuals

- ✦ Reduction in mortality due to early detection

❖ **Most Common Screening Methods**

- ✦ Mammography

- ✦ Clinical breast examination (CBE)

- ✦ Breast self-examination (BSE)

+ Table 4-1 shows the different guidelines for breast cancer screening of average-risk asymptomatic women.

❖ **Screening Mammography**

+ Currently, the most sensitive method for detecting early-stage breast cancer

+ Baseline mammogram

> *Begin by age 40 and then annually for average-risk asymptomatic women.*

TABLE 4-1
Guidelines for Screening Average-Risk Asymptomatic Women

Screening Technique	ACS[2]	NCI[3]
Breast self-examination	Monthly starting age 20	No recommendation
Clinical breast examination	20–39 years: every 3 years	No recommendation
	Annually start age 40	
Mammogram	Annually by age 40	Start by age 40
		Conduct every 1–2 years for women in their 40s who are at average risk
		Women at higher risk should consult physician about screening before age 40

ACS = American Cancer Society; NCI = National Cancer Institute.

Begin by age 25 for high-risk women or 5 years earlier than the earliest age when breast cancer was diagnosed in a family member.

Initiate yearly mammography in women with an identified genetic predisposition (BRCA1 and BRCA2 mutations).

✦ Benefits[4,5]

Reduction in mortality by 17% in asymptomatic women age 40 to 49

Reduction in mortality by 25% to 30% in asymptomatic women age 50 to 69

Smaller reduction in mortality for women over age 75

Detection of nonpalpable lesions that are correlated with a better prognosis

1. Twenty percent to 30% of nonpalpable lesions are found to be malignant at biopsy.

Greater than 85% sensitivity with mammography

✦ Limitations

Less effective in younger women due to breast tissue density

Cannot differentiate benign from malignant lesions

✦ Barriers to mammography

Lack of recommendation by primary care physician

False belief that having one mammogram is enough

False belief that mammograms are not required in the absence of symptoms

Underutilization pattern seen in older women and minorities

Lack of insurance coverage and costs of mammography

+ Prevalence of mammographic screening in 2000

58.5% among women age 40 to 64 years

60.8% among women age 65 and older

Table 4-2 shows the prevalence of mammography screening.

+ Racial and ethnic patterns in screening

Limited data are available about health behaviors and preventive health care services utilization among racial and ethnic minorities.

Proportion of African American women using

TABLE 4-2
Prevalence (%) of Mammographic Screening among U.S. Women[6]

Age at Mammogram	Median	Range
40–64	58.6	45.8–71.5
50 +	57.2	43.7–69.2
65 +	60.8	41.7–72.4

screening mammography is increasing and may be related to increased access and coverage through the Centers for Disease Control (CDC) National Breast and Cervical Cancer Early Detection Program.[6]

❖ Clinical Breast Examination

+ Recommended with every general physical examination

+ CBE every 3 years starting at age 20 to 39, according to ACS

+ Annually by age 40 in conjunction with mammography

+ Benefits of CBE

    Improves detection of breast cancer by 5% to 20%

+ Limitations of CBE

    Accuracy depends on the experience and skill of the examiner.

❖ Breast Self-Examination

+ Begin by age 20 and continue monthly, according to ACS.

+ May be the primary method of screening for young women who do not have regular CBE.

+ Benefits

    BSE helps increase breast health awareness.

Provides women with ability to understand anatomy and contour of breasts

Women need adequate instruction in learning how to perform BSE properly.

Low cost and low risk

+ Limitations

Anxiety and avoidance behaviors associated with performance of BSE

Lower sensitivity in detecting breast cancer compared with mammography

BSE is complementary to mammography and should not replace it.

❖ **Other Screening Tests**

+ Search for methods to increase accuracy of screening and to overcome barriers relating to film screen mammography.

+ Types

Digital mammography

Magnetic resonance imaging (MRI)

Positron emission tomography

Mammotome

Ultrasound

❖ **Digital Mammography**

+ Digital processing is a computerized tool for

capturing, enhancing, and storing mammographic images with the goal of increasing the accuracy of screening mammography, improving diagnosis, reducing the number of negative biopsies, and improving continuity of care.

+ The Food and Drug Administration (FDA) recently approved use of digital mammography.

+ Uses computer-aided digital displays and reduces time from imaging to display

+ Digital image can be manipulated, with adjustments for contrast and brightness.

+ Suspicious areas of concern can be magnified.

+ Benefits[1]

> *Image acquisition is fast because there is no film processing.*
>
> *Digital image can be manipulated to adjust for contrast and brightness.*
>
> *Regions of interest can be magnified.*
>
> *Computer video diagnosis and computer-aided detection (CAD) may decrease false-positive screening rates.*
>
> *May be useful in imaging dense breast tissue*
>
> *Decreases time required for breast compression*

+ Limitations

    Digital images must be viewed on specialized monitors that are very expensive.

    Brightness of specialized monitors is not equivalent to that of the traditional mammographic view box.

    Image manipulation may require more time for interpreting results.

    Full-field digital screening mammography units are costly.

❖ **Magnetic Resonance Imaging[7]**

+ Mammography lacks the specificity to separate benign from malignant lesions.

+ Increased interest in MRI to overcome problems of lack of mammographic specificity

+ Contrast agents tailored for use with MRI have improved sensitivity and specificity.

+ Contrast-enhanced imaging is based on the vascularity and vessel permeability difference between benign and malignant lesions.

    Benign conditions are poorly vascularized.

    Malignant lesions require vascular supplies.

+ Specific use of MRI

    Differentiates multifocal, multicentric, or diffuse masses

> *Sensitive in detecting small lesions less than 1 cm in size*
>
> *May be used when patients have very dense breasts.*

+ Benefits

> *Able to detect occult tumors that are not detected using mammography or CBE*

+ Limitations

> *Costly and invasive technique*
>
> *Must undergo quality assurance evaluation and standard setting similar to film-screen mammography*

❖ Positron Emission Tomography Scanning[8]

+ Procedure is based on the knowledge that malignant tumors use glucose more than does normal tissue.

+ When glucose is trapped in tumor cells, it allows imaging by means of positron emission tomography.

+ High specificity for malignancy

+ Sensitivity limited to tumors less than 8 mm

❖ Mammotome

+ Less time-consuming, nonsurgical procedure done under local anesthesia

+ Does not cause disfigurement

+ Safe to perform in women with breast implants

❖ **Ultrasound[9]**

+ Also called breast sonography

+ Ineffective as a screening method

+ Role is to evaluate specific areas of concern raised by mammography and CBE.

+ Uses

  Differentiate between cystic and solid palpable mass

  Evaluation of nonpalpable mass

+ Benefits

  Distinguishes solid from cystic mass

  Distinguishes between malignant and nonmalignant mass (e.g., abscess)

+ Limitations

  Expense

  Limited cost-benefit data

REFERENCES

1. Smith, R., & D'Orsi, C. (2000). Breast imaging and image-guided biopsy techniques. In J. R. Harris, M. Lippman, M. Morrow, & C. K. Osborne (Eds.), *Diseases of the breast* (2nd ed., pp. 101–121). Philadelphia: Lippincott Williams & Wilkins.

2. Smith, R., von Eschenbach, A., Wender, R., et al. (2001). American Cancer Society guidelines for the early detection of cancer. *CA: A Cancer Journal for Clinicians, 51,* 38–75.

3. National Cancer Institute. Statement from the National Cancer Institute on the National Cancer Advisory Board recommendation on mammography. (1997). Bethesda, MD: National Cancer Institute.

4. UK Trial of Early Detection of Breast Cancer Group. (1999). 16-year mortality from breast cancer in the UK trial of early detection of breast cancer. *Lancet, 353,* 1909–1914.

5. Hendrick, R., Smith, R., Rutledge, J., Smart, C. R. (1997). Benefit of screening mammography in women aged 40–49: A new meta-analysis of randomized controlled trials. *Journal of the National Cancer Institute Monograph, 22,* 87–92.

6. Smith, R., von Eschenbach, C., Wender, R., et al. (2001). American Cancer Society guidelines for the early detection of cancer. *CA: A Cancer Journal for Clinicians, 51,* 38–75.

7. Weinreb, J., & Newstead, G. (1995). MR imaging of the breast. *Radiology, 196,* 593–610.

8. Mautner, B., Schmidt, K., & Brennan, M. (2000). New diagnostic techniques and treatments for early breast cancer. *Seminars in Oncology Nursing, 16,* 185–196.

9. Kopans, D. (2000). Imaging analysis of breast lesions. In J. R. Harris, M. Lippman, M. Morrow, & C. K. Osborne (Eds.), *Diseases of the breast* (2nd ed., pp. 123–147). Philadelphia: Lippincott Williams & Wilkins.

5

Diagnosis and Staging

❖ Role of Clinical Breast Examination in Diagnosis

- ✦ Skin may show thickening, redness, dimpling, and/or inflammation.

- ✦ Changes in breast shape and variation in normal convexity may indicate an abnormality.

- ✦ Changes in appearance of nipple

    Retracted nipple looks flattened or pulled inward.

    Deviation of nipple shows change in the direction in which the nipple normally points.

    Thickening and loss of elasticity of the nipple may be a suspicious finding.

    Persistent scaly or eczema-like lesion may be an indication of Paget's disease.

- ✦ Characteristics of malignant breast nodule

    Usually a singular nodule

    Irregular or stellate shape

Firm or hard consistency

Fixed to skin or underlying tissues

Usually non-tender

Retraction may be present.

❖ Role of Mammography in Diagnosis

+ Bilateral mammography should be done before biopsy and will help determine

  Size of the suspicious mass

  Number of masses

  Baseline status

❖ Biopsy Techniques for Palpable Breast Masses

+ Techniques depend on the size and characteristics of the mass.

+ Types of biopsies for palpable masses

  Fine-needle aspiration (FNA)

  Fine-needle aspiration biopsy (FNAB)

  Core-needle or core-cutting biopsy

  Excisional biopsy

  Incisional biopsy

❖ Fine-Needle Aspiration and Fine-Needle Aspiration Biopsy

+ FNA and FNAB are complementary procedures

+ Used widely in Europe for many years

+ Gaining in popularity in the United States since the 1970s and 1980s

+ Procedure requires the skills of a cytopathologist

+ Advantages are several and include simplicity, good accuracy, low morbidity, minimal patient discomfort, low cost, and the immediate availability of an office procedure[1]

+ FNAB does not distinguish between invasive carcinoma and noninvasive ductal carcinoma in situ

❖ **Fine-Needle Aspiration**

  + Procedure

    Local anesthesia is generally not used because it requires a needle puncture.

    No. 21 1-in. needle is generally used for aspiration; size of the syringe varies from 3 to 10 mL.

    Typical cyst fluid is thin and opalescent; it varies in color from light tan to dark green.

    After aspiration, maintain pressure at the site for about 5 minutes to prevent bleeding into the cyst cavity.

  + Benign cystic mass disappears after aspiration.

  + Persistent residual mass, multiple recurrences after aspiration of the same cyst, and bloody aspirate indicate the need to obtain material for pathologic examination.

❖ Technique of Fine-Needle Aspiration Biopsy

✦ Procedure[1]

Skin is cleaned with an antiseptic.

If lesion is solid, a no. 25 needle may be used with a 20-mL syringe.

Needle is passed in and out of the lesion three to ten times in various directions.

Slight rotary motion allows the bevel of the needle to cut additional cells from the mass.

Appearance of aspirated material in the hub shows that an adequate amount of material is aspirated.

Suction on the plunger is released, and the needle and syringe are withdrawn.

Needle is disconnected from the syringe, and the syringe is filled with air.

Needle is replaced and a drop of material is placed onto a glass microscopic slide and spread with another slide.

Slides are wet-fixed or air-dried.

❖ Core-Cutting Needle Biopsy Technique

✦ Differs from FNA in that histologic material is obtained and does not require the skills of a cytopathologist.

✦ Core-cutting needle biopsies are processed for permanent or frozen sections.

+ Core-needle biopsies use disposable needles, such as Tru-Cut (Baxter Healthcare, Deerfield, IL) or a spring-loaded, core-cutting needle device.

  Tru-Cut needles are available at low cost.

  Spring-loaded devices have decreased pain associated with biopsy, better diagnostic sensitivity, and better specimen quality.

+ Advantages of core-cutting needle biopsy

  Better than excisional or incisional biopsy because it does not require open biopsy

  False-positive and false-negative rates are low.

  Possibility of seeding the needle track with tumor cells is low.

❖ Excisional Biopsy Technique

+ Complete removal of the tumor with a margin of surrounding normal tissue

+ Other interchangeable terms for excisional biopsy: *lumpectomy, tylectomy*

+ Definitive treatment for benign lesions

+ For malignant lesions, when a margin of surrounding normal tissue is removed and if pathologic examination confirms that the margins are clean of tumor, then no further breast surgery is needed.

+ Procedure

> *Performed under local anesthesia by a skilled surgeon*

> *When incisions are placed along Langer's lines (i.e., natural lines of skin tension and skin creasing), a better cosmetic result is obtained.*

> *When larger lesions are located in the lower half of the breast, a radial incision produces a better cosmetic result.*

> *Biopsy performed using a cold knife rather than electrocautery is preferred.*

> *If malignancy is suspected, lesions should be excised with a margin of normal surrounding tissue.*

❖ Incisional Biopsy Technique

+ Diagnostic biopsy that removes a portion of a mass for pathologic examination in cases in which complete removal is unnecessary or not possible

❖ Diagnosis of Non-palpable Lesions

+ Mammographic detection of small and non-palpable masses has resulted in an increased detection of earlier stage cancers leading to a 30% reduction in mortality.

❖ Excisional Biopsy of Non-palpable Lesions

+ Excisional biopsy after imaging-guided needle

localization is the gold standard for diagnosis of
lesions detected by mammography.[2]

✦ Advantage of excisional biopsy

> *Most accurate method of determining benign from
> malignant lesions*

✦ Pre-operative needle localization for surgical
excision

> *Several guides are used to assist the surgeon in
> resecting lesions that cannot be palpated.*
>
> *Guides rely on the positioning of a needle under
> imaging.*
>
> *Choice of guide depends on the surgeon and
> radiologist.*
>
> *Types of needle localization guides*
>
> 1. Hypodermic needle, hookwire, and
>   curved wires

✦ Methods used to guide needle localization and
biopsy

> *Ultrasound*
>
> 1. Used to guide biopsy or excision of
>   masses
>
> *Stereotactic mammography*
>
> 1. Used to guide biopsy of calcifications
>
> *Computed tomography*
>
> 1. Used when a lesion is visible on only one

mammographic view and not on any
other mammographic view

❖ **Image-Guided Percutaneous Biopsy of Non-palpable
Lesions**

✦ Image-guided percutaneous breast biopsy is an
acceptable alternative to open surgical biopsy.

✦ Advantages of image-guided percutaneous breast
biopsy

Procedure is well tolerated, fast, and inexpensive.

*Avoids the scarring and breast deformity associated
with open surgical biopsy*

Increasingly used in clinical practice

✦ Methods to diagnose image-guided biopsy for
non-palpable masses

FNA

Core-needle biopsy

✦ Both methods require imaging to guide needle
placement.[3]

*Stereotactic biopsy is used for lesions detected by a
mammogram.*

*Ultrasound is used for masses visualized by an
ultrasound.*

✦ Stereotactic biopsy

Two angled radiographic views acquired with the

x-ray beam at 15 degrees on either side of the center are used to determine the location of the lesion.

Computer algorithm uses geometric relations to calculate the position of the lesion based on the shift between the two acquired views.

Types of stereotactic biopsy units

1. Dedicated "prone" tables

2. "Add-on" adapted upright units

Dedicated prone table

1. Patient is placed in prone position on a specially designed table with opening, in which breast is suspended.

2. Breast is immobilized with compression plates and coordinates that can locate the non-palpable mass.

Add-on adapted upright unit

1. Less expensive and requires less space than a dedicated unit

2. Patient is seated and can see the biopsy.

3. Patient may experience more vasovagal reactions with the upright unit.

✦ Ultrasound

Used for masses that are sonographically evident

Advantages

1. Alternative to stereotactic core biopsy

2. Preferred by patients because there is no breast compression or radiation

Disadvantages

1. Difficulty in visualizing lesions such as small masses less than 6 mm, calcifications, or architectural distortions

❖ **Sentinel Lymphadenectomy or Sentinel Lymph Node Mapping**

✦ Definition: Removal of sentinel lymph node (first draining lymph node from tumor bed)

✦ When the sentinel lymph node is identified and when lymphatic drainage occurs in an organized pattern of progression, the sentinel lymph node reflects the pathologic status of the nodes.

✦ When the sentinel lymph node is biopsied and is pathologically free of cancer cells, then remaining nodes in the axilla are considered negative for cancer.

✦ Axillary node dissection may not be needed when the sentinel lymph node is negative.

❖ **Procedure**

✦ Blue dye is injected around the primary lesion and traced to the first blue node or sentinel node, or

+ Gamma probe mapping, using 99m Technetium-labeled sulfur colloid injected (radionuclide) preoperatively into the breast mass and then traced using a probe that is sensitive to gamma rays. Migration of radionuclide to the axilla is confirmed by lymphoscintigraphy and a gamma ray probe.

+ In combination with intraoperative lymphatic mapping, the procedure helps to decrease the risk associated with axillary node dissection (such as paresthesias, drains, immobility, cutaneous numbness, limited arm movement, fluid collection, and lymphedema).

❖ **Histologic Diagnosis**

+ Non-invasive carcinomas

  Ductal carcinoma in situ (DCIS)

  Lobular carcinoma in situ (LCIS)

+ Invasive carcinomas

  Infiltrating ductal carcinoma accounts for 75% of all invasive breast cancers.

  Infiltrating lobular carcinoma accounts for 5% to 10% of invasive breast cancers.

  Medullary carcinoma accounts for 5% to 7% of all invasive breast cancers.

  Mucinous and tubular carcinoma together account for about 5% of all invasive breast cancers.

+ Other Histology

  Inflammatory carcinoma

  Paget's disease (invasive or noninvasive)

❖ **Staging of Breast Cancer**

+ Staging of breast cancer is determined by the American Joint Committee on Cancer (AJCC).

+ AJCC system is a clinical and pathologic staging system based on the TNM classification (tumor, nodes, metastasis) (Table 5-1).

+ Clinical staging is based on physical examination.[4]

+ Pathologic staging is based on data used for clinical staging, surgical resection, and pathologic examination of the primary carcinoma.

+ Primary *tumor* is the size of the breast lesion.

+ *Nodes* refers to the involvement of regional lymph nodes.

+ Level I nodes (low axilla): Lymph nodes lateral to the lateral border of the pectoralis minor muscle

+ Level II nodes (mid-axilla): Lymph nodes between the medial and lateral borders of the pectoralis minor muscle and the interpectoral (Rotter's) lymph nodes

+ Level III (apical axilla): Lymph nodes medial to the medial margin of the pectoralis minor muscle, including those designated as subclavicular, infravicular, or apical

+ Internal mammary (ipsilateral): Lymph nodes in the intercostal spaces along the edge of the sternum in the endothoracic fascia

+ Other lymph nodes, including the supraclavicular, cervical, or contralateral internal mammary nodes, are coded as distant *metastasis.*

TABLE 5-1

TNM Classification and Staging of Breast Cancer[5]

Stage	Characteristics		
	Tumor (T)	Nodes (N)	Metastasis (M)
Stage 0	Carcinoma in situ or Paget's disease of nipple with no tumor	No regional lymph node involvement	No distant metastasis
Stage I	Tumor of 2 cm or less	No axillary node involvement	No distant metastasis
Stage IIA			
T0 N1 M0	No tumor	Movable ipsilateral axillary node involvement	No distant metastasis
T1 N1 M0	Tumor 2 cm or less	Movable ipsilateral axillary node involvement	No distant metastasis

TABLE 5-1
TNM Classification and Staging of Breast Cancer (*continued*)

Stage	Tumor (T)	Nodes (N)	Metastasis (M)
		Characteristics	
T2 N0 M0	Tumor 2–5 cm	No nodal involvement	No distant metastasis
Stage IIB			
T2 N1 M0	Tumor 2–5 cm	Movable ipsilateral axillary node involvement	No distant metastasis
T3 N0 M0	Tumor >5 cm	No nodal involvement	No distant metastasis
Stage IIIA			
T0 N2 M0	No tumor	Ipsilateral axillary lymph node(s) fixed to one another or to other structures	No distant metastasis
T1 N2 M0	Tumor <2 cm	Ipsilateral axillary nodes containing tumor growth and fixed to one another or other structures	No distant metastasis
T2 N2 M0	Tumor >2 cm but <5 cm	Ipsilateral axillary lymph nodes fixed to one another or to other structures	No distant metastasis
T3 N1 M0	Tumor >5 cm	Movable ipsilateral axillary node involvement	No distant metastasis

TABLE 5-1

TNM Classification and Staging of Breast Cancer (*continued*)

	Characteristics		
Stage	*Tumor (T)*	*Nodes (N)*	*Metastasis (M)*
T3 N2 M0	Tumor >5 cm	Ipsilateral axillary lymph nodes fixed to one another or to other structures	No metastasis
Stage IIIB			
T4 any N M0	Tumor of any size with direct extension to chest wall, peau d'orange or skin ulceration	With or without nodal involvement	No distant metastasis
Any T N4 M0	Tumor of any size	Metastasis to ipsilateral internal mammary lymph nodes	No distant metastasis
Stage IV			
	Tumor of any size with direct extension to chest wall or skin	Nodal involvement	Any metastasis

REFERENCES

1. Foster, R. (2000). Techniques of diagnosis of palpable breast masses. In J. Harris, M. Lippman, M. Morrow, & C. Osborne (Eds.), *Diseases of the breast* (2nd ed., pp. 95–100). Philadelphia: Lippincott Williams & Wilkins.

2. Kopans, D., & Smith, B. (2000). Preoperative imaging-guided needle localization and biopsy of nonpalpable breast lesions. In J. Harris, M. Lippman, M. Morrow, & C. Osborne (Eds.), *Diseases of the breast* (2nd ed., pp. 165–174). Philadelphia: Lippincott Williams & Wilkins.

3. Venta, L. (2000). Image-guided biopsy of nonpalpable breast lesions. In J. Harris, M. Lippman, M. Morrow, & C. Osborne (Eds.), *Diseases of the breast* (2nd ed., pp. 149–164). Philadelphia: Lippincott Williams & Wilkins.

4. Harris, J. (2000). Staging and natural history of breast cancer. In J. Harris, M. Lippman, M. Morrow, & C. Osborne (Eds.), *Diseases of the breast* (2nd ed., pp. 403–406). Philadelphia: Lippincott Williams & Wilkins.

5. American Joint Committee on Cancer: Breast. (1997). In *AJCC cancer staging manual* (5th ed., p. 171). Philadelphia: Lippincott–Raven.

PART II

Treatment of Primary Breast Cancer

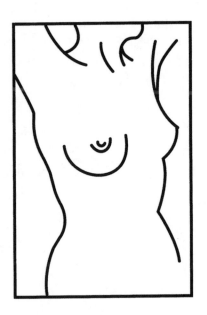

6

Surgical Techniques

❖ **Use of Surgery in Breast Cancer**

+ Treatment of non-invasive breast cancer

+ Modified radical mastectomy (MRM)

+ Total mastectomy

+ Breast conservation treatment (BCT)

+ Axillary lymph node dissection (ALND) or sampling

+ Sentinel lymph node biopsy (SLND)

❖ **Treatment of Non-invasive (In-Situ) Breast Cancer**

+ Aim of treatment is to prevent occurrence of invasive disease

+ Types of non-invasive breast cancer

Ductal carcinoma in situ (DCIS)

Lobular carcinoma in situ (LCIS)

❖ **Ductal Carcinoma in Situ**

+ With the widespread use of screening

mammography, 12% to 15% of breast cancers diagnosed annually are DCIS.[1]

+ Prior to screening mammography, DCIS was an unusual finding.

+ Microcalcifications are the most common mammographic finding in DCIS.

+ Linear and heterogeneous morphology is associated with cancer, while random calcifications throughout the breast are considered benign.

+ DCIS is a precursor with a variable risk of progression, depending on histology, lesion, size, and margins.

> *About 30% risk of invasive cancer at 10 years*
>
> *DCIS is associated with an excellent prognosis.*

+ Classifications of DCIS

> *Comedo*
>
> *Micropapillary*
>
> *Cribiform*
>
> *Solid*
>
> *Papillary*

+ Treatment of DCIS as primary diagnosis

> *Mastectomy is often recommended in the presence of extensive DCIS and microcalcifications.*

> *Breast-conserving surgery and radiation therapy*
> *plus tamoxifen is recommended for limited*
> *disease.*

✦ LCIS

> *Usually an incidental microscopic finding*
>
> *Considered a marker for breast cancer rather than*
> *premalignancy*
>
> *One percent increased risk of invasive disease per*
> *year*

✦ Surgical treatment

> *Observation due to the low risk of developing*
> *invasive carcinoma*
>
> *Bilateral prophylactic mastectomy with or without*
> *reconstruction has been used for patients*
> *unwilling to accept the risks associated with*
> *observation alone.*

❖ **Lobular Carcinoma In-Situ**

✦ LCIS is not detected on mammogram and is
  usually diagnosed by biopsy of a lesion.

✦ LCIS is associated with an increased risk of
  invasive breast cancer.

✦ LCIS was first described in 1941 as a noninvasive
  form of breast cancer that arises in the lobules and
  terminal ducts.

+ Lesion is usually an asymptomatic, incidental microscopic finding that does not show as a mass on mammography.

+ It is considered a risk factor or marker for breast cancer rather than a precursor.

  Seen more often in younger than older women

  LCIS is usually found on biopsy as a histologic component in pathologic specimens after surgery.

+ Current treatment for primary LCIS ranges from observation to bilateral mastectomy.

+ Because LCIS does not develop into invasive disease, it identifies women who are more likely to develop breast cancer; thus, they may be candidates for chemoprevention.

❖ **Follow-up in Patients with Non-invasive Breast Cancer[2]**

+ There is a risk of local recurrence or development of invasive breast cancer.

+ Recommendations based on National Comprehensive Cancer Network (NCCN) are semiannual physical examination and mammography.

❖ **Modified Radical Mastectomy for Primary Breast Cancer**

+ MRM is the most common surgical treatment for breast cancer in the United States.

+ Mastectomy as primary treatment reduces tumor mass and increases the effectiveness of systemic therapy.

+ Procedure

   Removal of the entire breast: nipple/areolar complex and pectoral fascia

   Level I, II, or III axillary lymph node dissection

   Pectoralis major is preserved

+ Indications for mastectomy

   Large, bulky tumors

   Multicentric disease

   Likelihood that the cosmetic outcome of breast-conserving surgery and radiation therapy may be poor.

   Patient preference and choice

❖ **Total Mastectomy**

+ Involves removal of the entire breast, with preservation of the pectoral muscles and axillary nodes

+ Candidates for total mastectomy

   Patients with DCIS

   Patients undergoing prophylactic mastectomy

   Patients who develop recurrence in the breast after breast-conserving surgery and radiation therapy

❖ **Complications of Mastectomy[3]**

✦ Wound infection

  Cellulitis in early postoperative period

  Abscess formation may occur as a late effect.

✦ Risk factors for infection

  Use of a two-step procedure with open biopsy and mastectomy

  Prolonged suction catheter drainage

✦ Necrosis of skin flaps is uncommon.

✦ Factors associated with necrosis of skin flaps

  Denuding subcutaneous fat from flap

  Closure of wound under tension

  Infection

  Occlusive pressure dressings

  Vertical incisions (currently not used)

✦ Phantom breast sensation

  About 50% of patients experience a residual sensation of the breast after mastectomy.

  Symptoms include pain, itching, nipple sensation, erotic sensation, and premenstrual-type soreness.

  Cause of phantom breast sensation is unknown, and symptoms may be constant over time.

❖ **Breast-Conserving Treatment**

+ BCT involves removal, wide excision of tumor and margin of normal surrounding tissue with preservation of the breast.

+ BCT and radiation therapy (XRT) is considered the standard treatment for most women with stage I and II breast cancer.[4]

+ Incidence of recurrence with BCT is 3% to 19%.

+ BCT treatment failure is treated with mastectomy.

+ No survival difference with BCT + XRT compared with mastectomy

+ Reader is referred to Chapter 8 for further information about treatment with XRT for primary breast cancer.

❖ **Axillary Lymph Node Dissection**

+ Number of involved axillary lymph nodes at diagnosis is one of the most important prognostic indicators in breast cancer.

+ Axillary lymph nodes are the major regional drainage site for the breast, receiving 85% of lymphatic drainage.

+ Likelihood that axillary nodes are involved with tumor is related to the size of the primary tumor, histologic grade, and presence of lymphatic invasion.

+ Axillary nodes are divided into three levels based on their anatomic relationship to the pectoralis minor muscle.

+ ALND is responsible for the major morbidity associated with breast cancer, including lymphedema, injury or thrombosis of the axillary vein, and injury to motor nerves in the axilla.

+ Other morbidity associated with ALND includes seroma formation, shoulder dysfunction, and loss of sensation in the distribution of the intercostobrachial nerve.

+ There is increased attention as to the value of ALND in women with early-stage primary breast cancer.

+ ALND may be considered an option in selected patients.

    Patients with favorable tumors

    Elderly patients

    Patients with serious concurrent morbidity

    Patients for whom selection of adjuvant therapy or hormonal therapy is not likely to be affected by evaluation of nodal status

❖ **Sentinel Lymph Node Biopsy**

+ Sentinel node is the first node that drains lymph from a cancer.[5]

+ If the sentinel lymph node is negative for the presence of malignancy, the rest of the axillary lymph nodes may be negative for disease.

+ Table 6-1 outlines the advantages and limitations of sentinel lymph node biopsy.

+ Technique involves the following:

> *Injection of Lymphazurin blue dye around the periphery of the primary tumor*
>
> *Breast massage to dilate the lymphatics*
>
> *Incision is made to search for the blue lymphatic channel leading to a blue-stained lymph node.*
>
> *Technique using a radiocolloid, such as technetium sulfur colloid, is less well established.*

TABLE 6-1

Advantages and Limitations of Sentinel Lymph Node Biopsy

Advantages of SLNB over ALND	*Limitations of SLNB*
Less invasive than level I–II axillary dissection	Possible false-negative results
May be more sensitive to detecting lymph node metastases	Not suitable for all patients (age and location of tumor limit success rate)
Potential to eliminate routine ALND for patients whose sentinel node is negative	Further technical improvements and studies are needed

+ Contraindications to SLNB include

    Palpable lymph node adenopathy

    Tumors larger than 5 cm in size or locally advanced breast cancer

    Use of preoperative chemotherapy

    Multifocal disease

    Prior major breast or axillary surgery that may interfere with lymphatic drainage

    Pregnant or lactating patient

❖ **Preoperative Patient Education**

+ Reinforce information and treatment recommendations.

+ Answer questions about hospital procedures, surgical experience, and follow-up home management.

+ Provide teaching materials, pamphlets, booklets, and websites dedicated to information about breast cancer and surgery.

❖ **Postmastectomy Nursing Care**

+ Because patients have a short length of inpatient stay, nursing care will concentrate on immediate postoperative care and teaching the patient self-care after discharge.

+ Major areas of focus for immediate postoperative care

Pain management

Monitor for hematoma, flap necrosis, and infection on day of surgery.

Assess the patient's psychosocial response.

+ Major areas of focus for self-care after discharge

+ Help the patient view the incisional site.

+ Teach the patient about incision care.

+ Examine the site for healing and prevention of infection.

+ Demonstrate how to empty and measure serous fluid from the drain, if present after discharge.

+ Demonstrate how to strip tubing and remove clots.

+ Provide a teaching pamphlet/booklet on exercises.

+ Discuss the importance of arm and hand exercises.

+ Discuss exercises to maintain range of motion.

+ Improve collateral circulation.

❖ **Postdischarge Patient Self-Care**

+ Patients must learn how to change the surgical dressing.

Manage surgical drains.

Monitor for signs of infection.

Continue hand and arm exercises 20 minutes a day, three times a week.

+ Maintain adequate nutritional and fluid intake to help healing of the incision.

+ Adapt home management techniques.

    Rest and relaxation

    Stress management

    Permit others to help with home, family, or work responsibilities.

+ Manage post-operative pain.

    Take prescribed medication.

    Assess for arm sensations (after axillary dissection).

    Assess for numbness, tingling, burning in axilla.

    Presence of arm sensations is normal.

❖ **Postdischarge Nursing Care Issues**

  + Review plans for the next step in cancer treatment and referral to

    Radiation therapy

    Chemotherapy and hormonal therapy

  + Review plans for surgical follow-up.

  + Assess the patient's psychosocial response.

  + Discuss whether the patient may be interested in accessing individual or support groups.

  + Suggest community resources for assistance.

  + Reinforce teaching and support for

Postmastectomy exercises

Lymphedema prevention

Management of fatigue

Help with body-image changes

Referral to prosthetist

REFERENCES

1. Winchester, D., & Goldschmidt, R. (2000). The diagnosis and management of ductal carcinoma in-situ of the breast. *CA: A Cancer Journal for Clinicians, 50,* 184–200.

2. Anderson, B., Bensinger, W., Cox, C., et al. (2000). NCCN practice guidelines for treatment of breast cancer. *Oncology, 14,* 33–49.

3. Morrow, M., & Harris, J. R. (2000). Primary treatment of invasive breast cancer. In J. R. Harris, M. Lippman, M. Morrow, & C. K. Osborne (Eds.), *Diseases of the breast* (2nd ed., pp. 515–560). Philadelphia: Lippincott Williams & Wilkins.

4. Giuliano, A. E., Jones, R. C., Brennan, M., et al. (1997). Sentinel lymphadenectomy in breast cancer. *Journal of Clinical Oncology, 15,* 2345–2350.

5. Hsueh, E., Hansen, N., & Giuliano, A. (2000). Intraoperative lymphatic mapping and sentinel lymph node dissection in breast cancer. *CA: Cancer Journal for Clinicians, 50,* 279–291.

7

Reconstructive Surgery

❖ Background

- ✦ Breast reconstruction has been used for the past 30 years, with many changes occurring in its development.

- ✦ About 150,000 reconstructive procedures for breast cancer are performed annually.[1]

❖ Breast Reconstruction

- ✦ Goals: Alleviate the deformity in the chest wall and breast after mastectomy.

- ✦ Considered an important part of cancer rehabilitation

- ✦ Challenges in reconstructive surgery today[2]

  Advances in flap design

  There is controversy over implant safety, due to which the U.S. Food and Drug Administration (FDA) placed a moratorium on the use of silicone gel implants, based on concerns over health risks.

The moratorium was lifted and patients with cancer who agree to participate in a clinical study are able to have saline implants.

New implant designs, including tissue expander and implant reconstruction, have overcome some of the barriers due to skin deficiency.

New methods of nipple reconstruction

Increased use of aggressive breast-conserving surgery requiring partial reconstruction

◆ Rationale for choosing breast reconstruction

Helps restore body symmetry

Helps decrease feelings of loss and disfigurement

Helps restore sense of femininity and sexuality

Helps to decrease reminder of breast cancer as a life-threatening illness

Improves ability to wear clothing

Decreases feelings of embarrassment about the prosthesis

Helps improve body image

◆ Reasons why women do not have breast reconstruction

Older age

Concern about a second surgical procedure

Uncertainty over the cosmetic outcome

Fear of discomfort and pain

Additional cost and expense

✦ What is the best breast reconstruction?

No single best procedure for all women

Decision about breast reconstruction and type is an individual one, based on risks and benefits.

✦ Timing of breast reconstruction

Immediate or delayed reconstruction is based on patient preference and choice.

Immediate reconstruction is performed in a majority of procedures today.

There are no differences noted in survival or recurrence rates with immediate or delayed reconstruction.

❖ **Immediate Reconstruction**

✦ Safe procedure that does not delay adjuvant therapy

✦ One surgical procedure is a cost-effective treatment.

✦ May help with body image adjustment and provide greater psychological benefit, compared with delayed reconstruction

✦ Federal laws in the United States require insurance companies to cover breast reconstruction after mastectomy.

❖ **Delayed Reconstruction**

- ✦ Gives patient time to adjust after the initial mastectomy procedure

- ✦ Provides patient with additional time to make an informed decision

- ✦ May be done up to several days to years after mastectomy

- ✦ Requires a second surgical procedure

- ✦ May result in a more visible scarring of the reconstructed breast

- ✦ Need for postoperative radiation may require delayed reconstruction.

- ✦ Table 7-1 outlines the technical consideration in using immediate or delayed reconstruction.

❖ **Types of Breast Reconstruction**

- ✦ Expander/implant

- ✦ Flap reconstruction

❖ **Expander/Implant**

- ✦ Tissue expansion, followed by removal of the expander and placement of the permanent implant, is the most common form of breast reconstruction in the United States because it provides an adequate reconstruction with the least amount of surgery.

- ✦ Procedure is recommended for women with small-

TABLE 7-1

Technical Considerations in Immediate and Delayed
Reconstruction

Immediate Reconstruction	Delayed Reconstruction
Less scar formation with stiffening and contracture	Mastopexy may be needed to achieve breast symmetry
Breast is more malleable	Tissue expander with delayed reconstruction allows skin to heal and decreases risk of mastectomy flap breakdown
Concurrent flap harvest during mastectomy, assisted elevation of mastectomy skin flaps help expedite procedure	Elevation of contracted, fibrotic skin flaps requires larger inset from the abdomen, leading to a less natural result
Preservation of inframammary fold and use of skin-sparing mastectomies help lead to a natural and symmetric reconstruction	

to moderate-sized breasts and little ptosis who
undergo a skin-sparing mastectomy.

+ Skin-sparing surgical techniques minimize skin
deficit.

+ Technical improvements in saline expanders and
implants that are contoured and textured have
improved the overall cosmetic outcome.

+ Implants do not match the natural shape and curve
of the natural breast.

Use of a bra or additional surgery on the opposite breast (e.g., reconstruction or breast augmentation) may lessen problems of achieving symmetry with implants.

+ Complications of the expander/implant are less than 10% in women who do not have postoperative radiation.

  Complications include infection, hematoma, extrusion, capsular contraction, pain, and deflation.

+ Choice of a saline versus a silicone gel implant for breast reconstruction depends on preference and choice (Table 7-2).

TABLE 7-2
Comparison between Saline and Silicone Gel Implants

Saline Implant	Silicone Gel Implant
Predominant choice over silicone gel	Available on investigational basis only
Firm and holds shape	Concern over link with connective tissue disorders, although studies do not demonstrate a relationship
Less likely to develop contracture	Softer and more natural feeling and texture
Contracture with silicone gel makes for a harder implant	Implant leakage and silicone gel bleed may occur over time

Reconstructive techniques have changed within the past 10 years. When silicone implants were placed in a single-stage procedure without tissue expansion, there was a higher risk of complications.

In patients with postoperative radiation, the complication rate may increase up to 18%.

+ Contraindications to expander/implant

Absolute contraindication is infection or lack of viable skin flap to close over the expander.

Relative contraindications include prior radiation, planned postoperative radiation, obesity, and smoking.

❖ **Flap Procedures**

+ Transverse rectus abdominus myocutaneous flap (TRAM flap)

+ Latissimus dorsi myocutaneous flap reconstruction

❖ **Transverse Rectus Abdominis Myocutaneous Flap**

+ TRAM is the major type of tissue reconstruction.

+ Procedure uses skin and fatty tissue from the lower abdomen to replace the skin (nipple and biopsy site) and breast tissue removed during mastectomy.

+ Rectus abdominis muscle is used as a conduit for

blood flow to overlying subcutaneous fat and skin of the lower abdomen.

+ TRAM flap replaces tissue lost with autologous tissue, which achieves a natural look and feel that is not possible with expander/implants.

+ TRAM is technologically complex and leaves a scar in the lower abdomen.

> *Patient must have adequate abdominal tissue, be a non-smoker, and be in generally good physical condition.*

+ Procedure can be initiated concurrently with mastectomy to reduce operative time.

+ Absolute contraindications to TRAM flap are prior upper abdominal incision with division of rectus abdominis and abdominoplasty.

+ Relative contraindications are older age, poor health, history of smoking, obesity, diabetes, hypertension, and thinness (e.g., not having enough lower abdominal tissue available for the procedure).

❖ **Free Transverse Rectus Abdominis Myocutaneous Breast Reconstruction**

+ Modification of the conventional TRAM flap to minimize problems of secondary blood supply and need for extensive dissection

+ Patients who may benefit from free TRAM include

smokers, the obese, and other high-risk patients, and patients requiring bilateral reconstruction.

+ This procedure offers the advantages of a reliable primary blood supply, limits dissection, and provides improved recovery after surgery.

+ Free TRAM is based on the deep inferior epigastric vessels, which are the primary blood supply to the lower abdomen.

+ Complications of free TRAM flap: Increase in potential for total flap loss around 3%, partial flap loss, and fat necrosis

❖ **Latissimus Dorsi Musculocutaneous Flap**

+ Less commonly used in comparison to the TRAM flap, but high patient satisfaction and low complications have increased the popularity of this procedure.

+ Alternative to TRAM for women with abdominal scarring or prior abdominal surgical procedures

+ Patients who have had prior radiation therapy have lower capsular contraction because the implants are covered by nonirradiated tissue.

+ Patients who require postoperative radiation after immediate reconstruction with the latissimus flap have a higher incidence of capsular contraction.

+ If a large amount of skin is removed, this procedure provides an excellent cosmetic result.

- ✦ Drawbacks: Skin color and texture may differ from that of the breast.

- ✦ Long-term results show that latissimus dorsi reconstruction is associated with high patient satisfaction, moderate capsular contracture rates, and minor flap loss.

- ✦ Implant infection rates are around 5%.

❖ Bilateral Free Transverse Rectus Abdominis Myocutaneous Flap

- ✦ Bilateral autologous reconstruction

- ✦ Procedure has been used for women having contralateral or prophylactic mastectomy.

- ✦ Women who have sequential mastectomies are not candidates for the TRAM flap.

- ✦ Bilateral pedicled TRAM breast reconstruction

  Requires sufficient lower abdominal tissue

  Procedure takes about 6 to 8 hours, and there is prolonged recovery.

  Associated with an increase in abdominal weakness

- ✦ In comparison, bilateral free TRAM flap reconstruction has advantages for patients who want to retain an active lifestyle and for high-risk patients.

  Flaps can be harvested at the same time as the mastectomy is performed.

> *Blood supply decreases fat necrosis and allows for better breast contouring.*

> *Vascularity of the upper abdominal skin flap is preserved because extensive tunneling is not needed.*

> *Benefits include good cosmetic outcome and lower abdominal morbidity.*

❖ Nipple–Areolar Reconstruction

- ✦ Nipple reconstruction helps to decrease the visual impact of a reconstructed breast.

- ✦ Without nipple reconstruction, there is no visual focal point other than the breast scar.

- ✦ Nipple reconstruction allows for a more natural-appearing "breast."

- ✦ Generally done after completion of reconstruction as a second-stage procedure in conjunction with mound revision or a contralateral symmetry procedure (e.g., breast reduction, mastopexy, or augmentation)

- ✦ Procedure may be done after completing adjuvant therapy.

- ✦ Areolar tattooing has provided better options over skin grafting.

- ✦ When needed, full-thickness skin grafts may be harvested from the groin or excess skin from the TRAM flap.

❖ **Nursing Management**

✦ Reconstruction minimizes the negative effects of breast cancer and treatment. Women choose reconstruction through a decision-making process of getting one's life back.[3]

✦ Teaching points

Reconstructed breast may approximate the look but will not look exactly like the former breast.

Patient may experience fewer sensations in the reconstructed breast.

✦ Post-surgical breast reconstruction nursing care

Prevention of infection

Pain management

Flap assessment: color, temperature, edema

Management of surgical wound

Prevention of seroma formation

Emotional support and body-image assessment

REFERENCES

1. Baker, R. (1992). The management of breast cancer with immediate or delayed reconstruction. *Advances in Surgery, 25,* 51–64.

2. Fine, N. A., Mustoe, T. A., & Fenner, G. (2000). Breast reconstruction. In J. R. Harris, M. Lippman,

M. Morrow, & C. K. Osborne (Eds.), *Diseases of the breast* (2nd ed., pp. 561–575). Philadelphia: Lippincott Williams & Wilkins.

3. Neill, K., Armstrong, N., & Burnett, C. (1998). Choosing reconstruction after mastectomy: A qualitative analysis. *Oncology Nursing Forum, 25,* 743–750.

8

Radiation Therapy

❖ Background

- ✦ In the 1900s, radiation therapy (XRT) was first used to treat patients with chest wall recurrence after surgery and as the primary treatment for patients with advanced breast cancer.

- ✦ Its role in the local management of breast cancer has changed significantly over the past hundred years.

❖ Uses of Radiation Therapy in Breast Cancer

- ✦ Primary local treatment in combination with breast-conserving surgery (BCS)

- ✦ Adjuvant-postoperative XRT

- ✦ Palliation (The reader is referred to Chapter 11 for further discussion.)

❖ Radiation Therapy for Primary Breast Cancer

- ✦ Increased percentage of early-stage disease with smaller primary tumors

- More breast-preserving options for women with early stage I and II breast cancers

- Improved radiation equipment, techniques, and procedures

- Wider availability of XRT facilities

- However, fewer than 50% of women with stage I and II breast cancer in the United States are treated with XRT.

- Benefits of XRT

    Improved cosmetic outcome

    Consideration of psychological and sexual concerns

    Equivalent to mastectomy for local control of disease[1]

- Contraindications to XRT[1]

    Patients who are in first and second trimester of pregnancy

    Two or more primary tumors in separate quadrants of the breast

    Diffuse microcalcifications within the breast

    Previous XRT to the same breast

    Persistent positive-tissue margins after surgery

- Relative contraindications

    History of collagen vascular disease (e.g., scleroderma, active lupus erythematosus)

    Multiple gross tumors in same breast quadrant

> *Presence of a large tumor in a small breast will limit the cosmetic outcome.*
>
> *Large breast size*

+ Goals of BCS and XRT

  > *Achieve survival equivalent to that of a mastectomy*
  >
  > *Maintain local control and low rate of recurrence in the breast*
  >
  > *Preserve cosmetic outcome for the patient*

+ Patient selection for XRT must take into account

  > *History and physical examination*
  >
  > *Mammographic evaluation*
  >
  > *Histologic assessment*
  >
  > *Patient needs and expectations*

+ Procedure

  > *BCS to excise gross tumor (e.g., excisional biopsy or lumpectomy) with clear margin of surrounding normal tissue*
  >
  > *Technical aspects related to lumpectomy include*

  1. Surgical incision directly over area of tumor

  2. Curvilinear or transverse incision when tumors are located in upper part of breast

  3. Preservation of subcutaneous fat and avoidance of skin flaps

Re-excision is indicated in the presence of positive tumor margins and unknown histologic margins of resection at initial surgery.

XRT to entire breast to eradicate microscopic residual disease

+ Risk factors for recurrence after BCS and XRT[1]

Young age is associated with increased risk of local recurrence and worse outcome after mastectomy.

Extensive intraductal component when margins of resection are not evaluated

Extent of resection using incisional biopsy is higher than with excisional biopsy.

Use of adjuvant systemic therapy decreases the rate of local recurrence.

❖ **Adjuvant Postoperative Radiation Therapy**

+ Postoperative XRT is the use of radiation to the chest and draining lymph nodes as adjuvant treatment after mastectomy.

+ Indications for use of postoperative radiation

Reduces rate of local–regional tumor recurrence (in chest wall, axilla, internal mammary or supraclavicular lymph nodes).

Improves survival by eradicating residual local disease that is the only site of persistent cancer after mastectomy and a potential source of distant metastasis or "seeding."

Improves survival by eradicating residual local disease that is the only site of persistent cancer after mastectomy and systemic therapy "reseeding."

+ Patients with four or more positive nodes or an advanced primary tumor benefit from postoperative XRT.[2]

+ XRT should not be given concurrently with anthracycline-containing chemotherapy.

+ XRT should be given within the first 6 months after mastectomy.

❖ Steps in the Radiation Treatment Process

+ Prior to starting radiation treatment, several steps must be completed.

+ Pretreatment consultation

Ideally, consultation occurs after diagnosis and before any local or systemic therapy is initiated.

A discussion of the specific role of XRT in the overall breast cancer treatment plan

During consultation, a physical examination is conducted, diagnostic studies are performed, and the radiation oncologist reviews the pathology.

+ Treatment planning

Once a decision is made to include XRT, the treatment planning session is initiated.

Treatment planning is also called a "simulation" procedure.

Goals of treatment planning are to maximize the radiation dose to the specific treatment area and minimize the dose to other normal tissues, such as lung and heart.

+ Treatment planning procedure

Takes approximately 1 hour

Radiation therapists and radiation oncologists measure the breast and axilla.

A series of x-rays are done on the simulation planning machine to delineate the breast and draining lymph node areas.

Skin surface markings are made to serve as landmarks for treatment.

Immobilization devices made of Styrofoam casts are made to help ensure consistent patient positioning for daily radiation treatments.

+ Patient teaching before treatment planning

The experience may appear frightening, impersonal, and uncomfortable.

Convey to the patient that the focus is on careful and detailed measurement.

Questions or concerns can be addressed before or after treatment planning.

*After treatment planning is complete, the patient
will receive an appointment to start daily XRT.*

❖ Daily Radiation Therapy Treatment

+ XRT consists of two components:

    External beam radiation to the primary tumor

    *Electron treatment or radiation implant to boost the
    site of the original tumor*

+ External beam radiation

    *High-energy photons emitted from a linear
    accelerator*

    *Radiation fields cover entire breast, the underlying
    chest wall, and the lower axilla, using opposing
    tangential fields to minimize lung and heart
    exposure*

    *A third anterior field may be added if the upper
    axillary and supraclavicular areas are included.*

    Whole-breast XRT dose ranges from 46 to 50 Gy.

    *Typical daily dose is 180 to 200 cGy delivered 5
    days a week over a 4.5- to 5-week period.*

+ Radiation boost to excision site

    *Goal is to increase local control to primary tumor
    site without decreasing cosmetic outcome.*

    Procedure

    1. Outpatient treatment after completion of
    XRT to whole breast

2. Electron beam penetrates tissue to a specific depth, allowing treatment of the tumor bed and sparing underlying lungs and ribs from radiation.

3. Treatment takes an additional five to eight daily fractions of 200 cGy.

4. Boosts total dose to the primary tumor site to 60 cGy or higher

✦ Radiation implant

Interstitial implantation of radioactive Iridium-192

Used as an alternative when boost treatment cannot be accomplished using electrons

1. Less frequently used method for radiation boost today

2. Invasive procedure requiring a 2- to 3-day hospital stay

✦ Nursing care during radiation implant

Manage mild discomfort associated with the procedure.

Reinforce necessity of radiation safety precautions for patient with nursing staff, family members, and visitors.

Provide emotional support to the patient during the isolation period.

❖ Patient and Family Education during Radiation Therapy[3]

+ Goals

Prepare the patient for the course of XRT.

Teach about potential side effects.

Help coordinate patient care activities during the radiation treatment experience.

+ Prepare for radiation treatment.

Describe the radiation treatment course—"Walk the patient through a treatment."

Explain the rationale for the total number of treatments needed and what patients can expect to hear and see in the treatment room.

Reassure the patient that she will not feel discomfort during the actual treatment.

Reassure the patient that radiation therapists will work closely with her during her therapy.

Time spent in radiation treatment room (15 minutes) is used to set up accurate positioning.

Actual treatment time is approximately 3 minutes.

❖ Side Effects of Radiation Therapy for Primary Breast Cancer

+ See Table 8-1.

TABLE 8-1
Potential Acute Side Effects of Radiation Therapy to Breast/Chest Wall

Side Effect	Average Onset	Usual Duration	Appearance/ Presentation	Intervention
Skin erythema	Approximately 2 weeks after start of treatment.	Resolution usually within 10 days to 2 weeks after end of treatment.	Variable. Mild redness to brisk or bright redness. Mild to moderate discomfort.	Unscented hydrophilic creams such as Aquaphor, Eucerin, Lubriderm. Unscented, 99–100% pure aloe vera gel (no added perfumes, colors). Avoid tight bras, underwire bras.
Hyperpigmentation	Approximately 2 weeks after start of treatment. May be more pronounced in darker pig-mented women.	Resolves slowly after end of treatment. Mild hyper-pigmentation may last for months.	Presents as mild to deep tanning of the skin. May be associated with mild discomfort.	As above
Itching/folliculitis (Irritation of hair follicles)	Approximately 10 days to 2 weeks after start of treatment.	Variable—may start to resolve at end of treatment course to entire breast (before start	Itchy skin appears slightly red and dry. Folliculitis appears as small red dots oftenin sternal,	Oatmeal colloidal based soaps (such as Aveeno). Make paste and apply to affected area, let dry for 3–5 minutes and rinse off with cool water. Oatmeal colloidal based bath

	Onset	Duration	Signs/Symptoms	Management
		of boost treatment); usually much improved by end of treatment course.	infraclavicular, and supraclavicular area. Occasionally found on back below clavicle 20 exit dose. May cause mild discomfort and itching.	products may be added to bath. 99–100% pure aloe vera gel (no added dyes or perfumes). Unscented hydrophilic creams such as those listed above for erythema. Diphenhydramine—25 mg may be taken at night for severe itching.
Fatigue	Highly variable approximately 2–3 weeks after start of treatment. May be an increased effect with previous or concurrent chemotherapy.	May last up to 2–3 weeks after end of radiation treatments. Average is 10 days to 2 weeks. May be prolonged if receiving chemotherapy.	Increased tiredness late afternoon or early evening. Most women are able to continue their usual routines.	Earlier bedtime, late afternoon or early evening rest period. Good nutrition—avoid dieting during course of treatment. Conserve energy by having family and friends help as needed. Moderate exercise such as walking has been found to help energy levels.
Dry desquamation (dry peeling)	Approximately 3 weeks after starting radiation.	Usually resolves within 2 weeks of finishing radiation treatments.	Dry flaking or peeling of skin frequently associated with erythema or hyperpigmentation of skin.	Use of highly moisturizing hydrophilic creams such as Aquaphor and Eucerin.

continued

TABLE 8-1
Potential Acute Side Effects of Radiation Therapy to Breast/Chest Wall *(continued)*

Side Effect	Average Onset	Usual Duration	Appearance/ Presentation	Intervention
Moist desquamation (moist peeling)	4–5 weeks after start of radiation therapy.	Usually completely healed within 2–3 weeks after end of radiation treatments.	Moist peeling of the skin with associated erythema. Area may ooze or weep. May be associated with mild to moderate discomfort depending on severity of reaction. Increased reaction is possible if patient receiving concurrent chemotherapy. Often occurs in areas with increased shearing	Gentle rinsing with drying anti-bacterial solutions such as Hibiclens/ chlorhexidine gluconate or $1/4$–$1/2$ strength H2O2. Pat dry with soft clean towel 2–3 times a day.

Above can be followed by application of unscented hydrophilic cream such as Aquaphor, followed by non-adherent dressing such as Aquaphor gauze, covered with a soft ABD pad and held in place by a bra or large size body netting.

Moist soaks can be used such as aluminum acetate solutions: Bluboro and Domeboro for 20 minutes 3 times a day. |

			friction such as inframammary fold and axilla.	Moisture vapor permeable dressing may be used such as Op-site, although they can be difficult to adhere in skin folds.
				Avoid use of tape on irritated skin.
				Can use gentle lukewarm shower spray to help debride skin.
				Allow area to be open to air whenever possible.
				If pain is moderate or severe use of NSAID, or mild narcotic may be indicated.
Intermittent aches and pains in breast	May occur approximately 1 week after start of radiation.	Can persist for months after radiation finishes although usually with decreased frequency.	Patients often describe pain as intermittent sharp twinge in the breast.	Reassurance that this is a normal occurrence and may be alleviated with use of NSAID.

continued

TABLE 8-1
Potential Acute Side Effects of Radiation Therapy to Breast/Chest Wall *(continued)*

Side Effect	Average Onset	Usual Duration	Appearance/ Presentation	Intervention
Breast edema	As above.	Can persist for months after radiation.	Slight to moderate swelling of treated breast. Breast may feel full or heavy.	As above. Wearing a supportive bra may improve comfort.
Hair loss in treatment portal (fine hair of breast, nipple, and possibly small amount of axillary hair)	Usually starts 3–4 weeks at doses of 30–35 Gy.	Variable. May take 1–6 months for hair to grow back.	Typically not very noticeable or bothersome to patients except when associated with folliculitis or itching.	Follow interventions for itching/ folliculitis.

Source: Karen Hassey Dow, *Contemporary Issues in Breast Cancer,* 1998, Sudbury, MA: Jones and Bartlett Publishers. www.jbpub.com. Reprinted with permission.

+ Acute and late effects

> *Acute side effects occur during treatment and up to 6 months post-XRT.*

> *Late effects occur after 6 months (reader is referred to Chapter 14 for a discussion of late effects of XRT).*

+ Common acute side effects

> *Skin reactions*

> *Arm and breast edema*

> *Intermittent aches and pains in the treated breast, chest wall, or axilla*

> *Fatigue*

+ Teaching points about side effects

> *Emphasize local versus systemic effects of XRT.*

> *Reassure patients that they will not become radioactive.*

> *Teach patients that they will not experience severe skin "burns."*

> *Clarify information, dispel misconceptions, and identify fears about radiation as a treatment modality.*

❖ **Skin Reactions**[4,5]

+ Erythema or redness

May occur immediately after first radiation treatment

This skin reaction is generally dose-dependent and increases throughout the course of XRT.

Fair-skinned individuals are at higher risk.

Increase in redness is also heightened along a bony prominence, such as the clavicle.

+ Increased pigmentation

Skin reaction is dose-dependent and most often occurs in darker pigmented individuals.

Pigmentation appears as series of dark dots in the treatment field.

+ Folliculitis with pruritus

Skin reaction is dose-dependent.

Mild emollient or lotion will help decrease itchiness.

Oatmeal-based soap applied to the skin may help relieve itchiness.

Areas of higher risk include the skin folds and general breast area.

+ Hair loss in the treated area

Reaction is temporary.

+ Dry desquamation (dry peeling)

   Most commonly seen in areas of bony prominence, such as the clavicle

   Mild emollient placed on the skin after treatment will help soothe the irritated area.

+ Moist desquamation (moist peeling)

   Skin reaction is dose-dependent and most often occurs with concurrent chemotherapy.

   Rarely occurs without concurrent chemotherapy

   Several skin-care guidelines are available to manage moist reactions.

   May require a radiation treatment break if the moist reaction is severe

+ Factors influencing skin reactions

   Skin folds (i.e., inframammary and axilla) included in the radiation treatment field

   Older age

   Concurrent use of topical steroids near the XRT field

   Higher radiation dose fraction and higher total radiation dose

   Enhanced skin effects in electron beam boost

   Enhanced skin reactions, with chest wall radiation occurring at the XRT beam exit site in the upper back

+ Management of skin reactions[6]

  Majority of skin-care regimens for patients receiving breast irradiation are non-research based.

  Recommendations depend on what has worked most effectively in clinical practice and on institutional policies (Table 8-2).

❖ **Arm and Breast Edema**

  + Arm edema or lymphedema occurs most often in patients receiving XRT to the axilla after axillary dissection.

  + Etiology is not well understood but is related to obliteration of lymphatics in the axilla by surgery and XRT.

  + Reader is referred to Chapter 16 for a more detailed discussion about lymphedema.

  + Breast edema occurs as mild breast discomfort and feelings of fullness in the treated breast.

  + Arm and breast edema may occur shortly after radiation is complete or within the first year after XRT.

  + Breast edema may take up to several months to resolve.

    Breast edema may be treated with nonsteroidal anti-inflammatory drugs.

    Symptomatic relief using cotton sport bras helps alleviate heaviness and discomfort.

TABLE 8-2

General Skin-Care Guidelines for Radiation Treatment to the Breast/Chest Wall

General skin-care guidelines are provided to patients at the beginning of the course of radiation and are as follows:

1. Keep breast or chest wall clean and dry

2. Cleanse the treated area with gentle soap (e.g., Ivory, Basis, Pears, Neutrogena, or unscented Dove)

3. Avoid the use of creams, lotions, perfumes, or deodorant in the treatment area unless directed by a radiation oncologist, nurse, or radiation therapist

4. Avoid extremes of temperature, such as heating pads, hot-water bottles, and ice packs in the treatment area. Avoid Jacuzzis and saunas

5. Avoid excess friction or rubbing

6. Do not use tight clothing or underwire bra; use sports bra during XRT

7. Use an electric razor to shave under the treated arm

8. Protect the skin in the treatment field from exposure to direct sunlight by either covering the skin or using a sunblock with SPF of 15 or higher

Aftercare

General aftercare instructions include the following:

1. Occasional aches and pains in the treated breast/chest wall may continue for weeks or months after finishing XRT. Use an NSAID such as ibuprofen

2. Skin changes will gradually improve over the 1 to 2 weeks following completion of treatment. The treated skin may look tanned

TABLE 8-2
General Skin-Care Guidelines for Radiation Treatment to the Breast/Chest Wall (*continued*)

3. The breast tissue may feel thicker and firmer after XRT. Continue self-breast examinations monthly in order to remain familiar with the feel of the breast tissue

4. Call oncology team with any concerns or questions

5. The skin may feel dry after radiation therapy. Use a skin moisturizer for at least 2 weeks after the end of radiation treatment

6. If previously irradiated skin is exposed to direct sunlight, cover or protect with SPF 15 or higher

7. If you develop any areas of redness, heat, or swelling in the treated breast, hand, or arm, call your health care provider

The following information should be included if patients have had an axillary dissection and/or XRT to the axilla

8. Wear gloves when gardening or using harsh chemicals such as bleach

9. For a long period of time, avoid using the affected arm/hand to carry heavy packages

10. If you get a cut or burn on the affected arm/hand, gently cleanse the area and apply antibacterial cream

11. Use the untreated arm for blood drawing, blood pressures, and vaccinations and/or injections

---

❖ Intermittent Twinges and Shooting Pains

- ✦ Occur in treated breast, chest wall, or axilla

- ✦ Common and normal after surgery and radiation therapy

+ Treat with mild analgesics.

+ Twinges may last for several months to years after treatment ends.

❖ **Fatigue**

+ Very common reaction experienced by patients receiving XRT

+ Mechanisms of radiation-related fatigue are not well understood.

+ Most likely a multifactorial etiology

   Recovery from recent surgery

   Previous or concurrent chemotherapy

   Increased tumor burden

   Concurrent medications, such as antiemetics or analgesics, may increase drowsiness.

   Nutritional deficit

   Demands of daily treatment in the radiation oncology department for a period of 5 to 6 weeks may tax energy levels.

   No corresponding decrease in family and work responsibilities during XRT may increase energy demands.

   Presence of other symptom clusters, such as sleeplessness and restlessness and anxiety over disease and treatment

*Interventions for fatigue—Reader is referred to
Chapter 15 for further discussion of cancer-
related fatigue.*

❖ Emotional Response during Radiation Therapy

+ Patients may experience many emotional reactions
  during the course of XRT. Emotional reactions may
  not necessarily be related directly to radiation but
  to the experience of having breast cancer. In
  addition, there may be an age-related emotional
  response to treatment.[7] Thus, it is important for
  the radiation oncology nurse to

  *Assess patient's psychosocial status before treatment
  and regularly during XRT*

  *Suggest availability of support groups, discussion
  groups, and community resources, and refer as
  needed*

  Discuss other psychosocial interventions available[8]

  *Provide a number for patients to call and speak
  directly to a nurse for questions or concerns*

REFERENCES

1. Morrow, M., & Harris, J. R. (2000). Primary treatment of
   invasive breast cancer. In J. R. Harris, M. Lippman,
   M. Morrow, & C. K. Osborne (Eds.), *Diseases of the breast*
   (2nd ed., pp. 515–560). Philadelphia: Lippincott
   Williams & Wilkins.

2. National Institutes of Health. NIH Consensus Development Conference Statement on Adjuvant Therapy for Breast Cancer, November 1–3, 2000. Available online at: http://consensus.nih.gov

3. O'Rourke, N., & Robinson, L. (1996). Breast cancer and the role of radiation therapy. In K. H. Dow (Ed.), *Contemporary issues in breast cancer* (pp. 43–58). Sudbury, MA: Jones and Bartlett.

4. Sitton, E. (1992). Early and late radiation-induced skin alterations Part I: Mechanisms of skin changes. *Oncology Nursing Forum, 19,* 801–807.

5. Porock, D., Kristjanson, L., Nikoletti, S., et al. (1998). Predicting the severity of radiation skin reactions in women with breast cancer. *Oncology Nursing Forum, 25,* 1019–1029.

6. Sitton, E. (1992). Early and late radiation induced skin alterations Part II: Nursing care of irradiated skin. *Oncology Nursing Forum, 25,* 907–912.

7. Dow, K., & Lafferty, P. (2000). Quality of life, survivorship, and psychosocial adjustment of young women with breast cancer after breast-conserving surgery and radiation therapy. *Oncology Nursing Forum, 27,* 1555–1564.

8. Kolcaba, K., & Fox, C. (1999). The effects of guided imagery on comfort of women with early stage breast cancer undergoing radiation therapy. *Oncology Nursing Forum, 26,* 67–72.

9

Adjuvant Therapy, Targeted Therapy, and Hormonal Therapy in Primary Breast Cancer

✦ Adjuvant chemotherapy is defined as the administration of cytotoxic chemotherapy or the use of ablative or additive endocrine therapy after primary surgery of breast cancer to kill or inhibit clinically occult micrometastases.[1]

❖ **Prognostic and Predictive Factors Used to Select Adjuvant Chemotherapy**

✦ Several prognostic and predictive factors are used to help identify patients who may benefit from adjuvant chemotherapy. The factors are outlined in Tables 9-2 and 9-3.

✦ Guidelines for treatment of breast cancer have been developed by the National Comprehensive Cancer Network (NCCN) in conjunction with the

American Cancer Society and can be accessed at: http://www.nccn.org/patient_guidelines/ breast_cancer/breast/1_introduction.htm

✦ The rapid pace of discovery in the development

TABLE 9-1

Historical Perspective in the Use of Adjuvant Chemotherapy

1960–1970s	Postoperative adjuvant chemotherapy used in patients with involved lymph nodes
Mid-1970s	Tamoxifen as adjuvant hormonal therapy started
1980s	Doxorubicin-based chemotherapy trials Clinical trials chemotherapy in patients without axillary nodal involvement Combined chemoendocrine therapy
1990s	High-dose chemotherapy with autologous bone marrow transplantation Neoadjuvant chemotherapy Taxanes in adjuvant trials

TABLE 9-2

Accepted Prognostic and Predictive Factors[1]

Patient characteristics	Age Race (prognostic factor only)
Disease characteristics	Tumor Size (T) Histologic tumor type Axillary nodal status (N) Pathologic Grade
Biomarkers	Hormone receptor status Mitotic rate

TABLE 9-3
Promising Prognostic and Predictive Factors

Tissue and expression microarrays	HER2
Proteomics	p53 status
Sentinel lymph node biopsy	Histologic evidence of vascular invasion
Assays for micrometastatic disease	Quantitative parameters of angiogenesis

of new therapies continues to expand the knowledge base from which informed treatment decisions can be made. Thus, the National Institutes of Health convened a Consensus Development Conference for the purpose of establishing consensus regarding the use of adjuvant therapy for invasive breast cancer. The statement is based on the relevant literature, presentations, and audience discussion. The following is a summary of the Conference statement:

❖ **Summary of NIH Consensus Development Conference Statement on Adjuvant Therapy for Breast Cancer[2]**

✦ Chemotherapy can significantly improve the duration of relapse-free and overall survival in both premenopausal and postmenopausal women up to age 70 years with node-positive and node-negative disease.

+ Indication for adjuvant polychemotherapy is for breast cancers larger than 1 cm in diameter regardless of nodal, menopausal, or hormonal status

+ Anthracycline-containing regimens (e.g., doxorubicin and epirubicin) show a small but statistically significant improvement in survival compared with nonanthracycline-containing regimens.

+ Dose-dense chemotherapy regimens (e.g., high-dose chemotherapy with peripheral stem cell support) have not resulted in improved survival outcomes compared with standard polychemotherapy, and thus should be offered within a randomized clinical trial.

+ Taxanes (e.g., paclitaxel and docetaxel) are being investigated in the adjuvant treatment of node-*positive*, localized breast cancer.

+ Taxanes in women with node-*negative* breast cancer should be restricted to randomized clinical trials.

❖ **Adjuvant Chemotherapy Regimens**

+ Polychemotherapy with two or more agents has been shown to be superior to single-agent chemotherapy.

+ Anthracycline-containing adjuvant chemotherapy regimens (e.g., doxorubicin or epirubicin) have shown a statistically significant survival advantage compared with non-anthracycline containing regimens.

+ Four to six courses of treatment provide optimal benefit.

   More than six months of chemotherapy does not improve overall outcome.

+ Threshold dose effects have been demonstrated with doxorubicin (A) 60 mg/m^2 and cyclophosphamide (C) 600 mg/m^2.

+ AC has not been compared with cyclophosphamide, doxorubicin, fluorouracil (CAF) or cyclophosphamide, epirubicin, or fluorouracil (CEF) in a randomized clinical trial.

+ Results of several clinical trials show that four cycles of anthracycline-containing regimens that consist of AC or EC (epirubicin/ cyclophosphamide) are equivalent to cyclophosphamide, methotrexate, fluorouracil (CMF)

+ Anthracycline-containing regimens of three or more drugs (e.g., CAF, CEF, fluorouracil, epirubicin, or cyclophosphamide [FEC]) have been shown superior to CMF in terms of relapse-free survival.

+ No evidence for excessive cardiac toxicity in women without significant preexisting heart disease treated with anthracyclines using the cumulative doses in standard adjuvant chemotherapy regimens[3]

❖ **Taxanes in the Adjuvant Setting[4]**

+ Paclitaxel was the first taxane that proved to be effective in the treatment of metastatic breast cancer.[5,6]

+ Two generations of adjuvant pivotal trials with taxanes include:

> *Comparison of taxane/anthracycline regimen with non-taxane combinations or sequence regimens*

> *Comparison of taxanes in both arms comparing their use in combination or in sequence*

+ Cancer and Leukemia Group B (CALGB-9344) randomized 3,170 patients with node positive breast cancer to a fixed dose of cyclophosphamide (600 mg/m^2) plus doxorubicin at 60, 75, or 90 mg/m^2, followed by second randomization to either four doses of paclitaxel 175 mg/m^2 or no further chemotherapy.

> *The sequential use of AC plus paclitaxel improved odds of recurrence-free and overall survival by more than 20% when compared with AC alone[7]*

> *Doxorubicin dose escalation higher than 60 mg/m^2 had no impact on disease-free survival.[8]*

+ Early results led to Federal Drug Administration (FDA) approval of paclitaxel following four cycles of AC (anthracycline + cyclophosphamide) in the adjuvant setting.

+ AC with or without sequential paclitaxel has evolved as standard chemotherapy in node-positive breast cancers. While the benefit in node–positive patients is clear, the role in node-negative patients has yet to be clearly elucidated. The National Surgical Adjuvant Breast and Bowel Project (NSABP) B-28 study should clarify this matter.

+ CALGB-9741 continues to further explore clinical benefit by comparing a three-weekly regimen of AC followed by paclitaxel with a two-weekly, dose-dense regimen using the same drugs with G-CSF support.

+ Breast Cancer International Research Group (BCIRG) is evaluating the effectiveness taxanes by randomizing patients to either six cycles of AC + docetaxel 75 mg/m^2 or AC + 5 FU 500 mg/m^2.[9]

❖ Adjuvant Chemotherapy

+ Table 9-4 outlines chemotherapy commonly used for breast cancer and includes: cyclophosphamide, doxorubicin, epirubicin, paclitaxel, docetaxel, 5-fluorouracil, and methotrexate.

TABLE 9-4
Adjuvant Chemotherapy

Cyclophosphamide (Cytoxan)

Mechanism of action	Alkylating agent that causes cross-linking of DNA strands that prevent DNA synthesis and cell division
Indications/Use	Adjuvant therapy
Range of dosage	600 mg/m^2 IV every three weeks 100 mg/m^2 PO on days 1–14 of a 28-day cycle
Special precautions	
Toxicity	Nausea and vomiting Alopecia Urotoxicity, hemorrhagic cystitis Myelosuppression

Doxorubicin

Mechanism of action	Anti-tumor antibiotic that binds directly to DNA base pairs and inhibits DNA and RNA synthesis
Indications/Use	Adjuvant therapy Advanced disease
Range of dosage	60–75 mg/m^2 IV every 21 days 30 mg/m^2 IV day 1 and 8 of 28-day cycle
Special precautions	Maximum cumulative lifetime dose is 550 mg/m^2 <400 mg/m^2 cumulative lifetime dose recommended in patients who have had prior cardiotoxic regimens or chest radiation Vesicant
Toxicity	Cardiotoxicity Nausea and vomiting Myelosuppression Alopecia Stomatitis

TABLE 9-4
Adjuvant Chemotherapy (*continued*)

Epirubicin (EPI)

Mechanism of action	DNA strand breakage mediated by anthracycline effects on topoisomerase II
Indications/Use	Advanced disease
Range of dosage	70–90 mg/m^2 IV every 3 weeks
Special precautions	Vesicant
	Administer through sidearm of freely flowing IV infusion
	Lifetime cumulative dose of 900–1000 mg/m^2
	Reduce dose in patients with prior chest radiation or anthracycline
Toxicity	Myelosuppression: dose limiting leukopenia
	Nausea and vomiting: common
	Stomatitis: dose-dependent
	Alopecia
	Cardiac effects: potentially irreversible congestive heart failure
	Red orange discoloration of urine
	Diarrhea: occasional

Paclitaxel (TAXOL)

Mechanism of action	Taxane
	Enhanced formation and stabilization of microtubules
Indications/Use	Adjuvant therapy
	First and second line-chemotherapy for metastatic disease
Range of dosage	175 mg/m^2 as 3-hour infusion every 3 weeks
	80–100 mg/m^2 as a 1-hour infusion every week
Special precautions	Hypersensitivity reaction minimized with pretreatment of: dexamethasone 20 mg orally or intravenously 12 hours and 6 hours prior

TABLE 9-4
Adjuvant Chemotherapy (*continued*)

	to infusion, diphenhydramine 50 mg IV and cimetidine 300 mg IV 30 minutes prior to infusion
	Mixed in containers that do NOT contain polyvinylchloride or diethylhexlphtalate (DEHP) plastics
	Use an in-line filter
	Do not administer if patient has known sensitivity to Cremophor EL
	ANC should be >1500 prior to initial or subsequent doses of paclitaxel
	Avoid concomitant use of ketoconazole
	Cardiac monitoring if history of conduction abnormalities
	First hour of infusion, take vital signs every 15 minutes; second hour of infusion, take vital signs every 30 minutes; or per hospital policy
Toxicity	Dose-limiting: neutropenia, mucositis (with longer infusion), neurotoxicity
	Frequent: myalgias, arthralgias, alopecia
	Rare: thrombocytopenia, anemia, nausea and vomiting, diarrhea
	Hypersensitivity reaction (dyspnea, hypotension, bronchospasm, urticaria may result from Cremophor)
5-fluorouracil	
Mechanism of action	Pyrimidine antimetabolite; inhibit the formation of thymidine synthetase needed for DNA synthesis.
Indications/Use	Adjuvant therapy
Range of dosage	500–600 mg/m² IV
Special precautions	

TABLE 9-4
Adjuvant Chemotherapy (*continued*)

Toxicity	Neutropenia and thrombocytopenia
	Cutaneous effects in nails, skin, hair loss
	Nausea and vomiting

Methotrexate

Mechanism of action	Antimetabolite, folic acid antagonist; blocks the enzyme dihyrofolate reductase that inhibits conversion of folic acid to tetrahydrofolic acid. Inhibits precursors of DNA, RNA, and cellular proteins
Indications/Use	Adjuvant therapy
Range of dosage	40 mg/m^2 IV days 1 and 8 of 28-day cycle
	40 mg/m^2 IV day 1 of 21-day cycle
Special precautions	
Toxicity	Stomatitis
	Diarrhea
	Nausea and vomiting

Docetaxel (Taxotere)

Mechanism of action	Inhibits mitotic spindle apparatus by enhanced formation and stabilization of microtubules
Range of dosage	60–100 mg/m^2 as a 1 hour infusion every 3 weeks
Special precautions	Severe hypersensitivity reactions (flushing, hypotension, dyspnea) can be minimized with premedication of dexamethasone 8 mg PO BID for 5 days starting 1 day before docetaxel
	Should not infuse through polyvinyl chloride (PVC) tubing
Toxicity	Myelosuppression common and dose-limiting
	Hypersensitivity reaction uncommon

TABLE 9-4
Adjuvant Chemotherapy (*continued*)

Alopecia, skin and nail changes
Nausea and vomiting: common and brief
Mild mucositis
Fluid retention common
Fatigue, myalgias common
Mild sensorimotor neuropathy

❖ Optimal Sequencing of Adjuvant Chemotherapy

✦ Perioperative adjuvant chemotherapy

Potential benefit is that chemotherapy given at the time of or just after surgery may kill circulating tumor cells that may be dislodged at the time of surgery.

After removal of primary tumor, DNA synthesis and proliferation of distant micrometastasis increase and thereby may increase their vulnerability to cytotoxic drugs.

Immediate treatment may limit drug resistance.

Meta-analysis of perioperative trials showed a modest improvement in disease-free survival but not overall survival benefit and thus, the use of perioperative chemotherapy is limited.

✦ Neoadjuvant chemotherapy

Administering chemotherapy before surgery helps

> to assess sensitivity and response of a tumor to chemotherapy.

> Early detection of a resistant tumor can help avoid unnecessary toxicity with drugs that are of little or no benefit.

> The earlier the disease is treated, the less potential for drug resistance.

> Large tumors can be shrunk to allow breast-preserving surgery rather than mastectomy.

> Neoadjuvant chemotherapy has been used in patients with inoperable, locally advanced breast cancer with tumors larger than 3 cm.

> Limitations: control of distant micrometastasis is not improved, staging of axilla is a problem, pretreatment of molecular markers is more difficult

❖ **Support for Decision-Making in Adjuvant Chemotherapy[2]**

✦ Patients need time to discuss and share their concerns in making decisions about chemotherapy. Effective communication between the oncology team and the patient is critical. The following are points to consider in helping to support patients in their decision-making:

> Clarify their concerns and help evaluate risks and benefits with treatment.

Discuss how treatment may alter lifestyle and daily routines.

Explain the range treatment side effects and management.

Explore impact of treatment on their personal quality of life.

Discuss their concerns about clinical trials.

+ The Department of Defense Breast Cancer Decision Guide includes an interactive consultation to help women in the decision-making process and can be accessed at: http://bcdg.org

❖ Promising New Research for Adjuvant Chemotherapy[2]

+ Given the changes in treatment and the promise of new strategies that combine chemotherapy and targeted, novel therapies, the Consensus Development Panel recommended the following avenues of research:

Randomized clinical trials to further evaluate the role of taxanes and high-dose chemotherapy

Evaluating the importance of variations in the dose and schedules of currently used adjuvant chemotherapy

Clinical trials to determine the clinical and biological characteristics for accurately predicting the effectiveness of specific adjuvant treatments in individualized patients

Trials to determine the effectiveness of adjuvant chemotherapy in patients older than 70 years

+ In addition, PDQ at the National Cancer Institute can be accessed for the latest information on breast cancer and clinical trials at http://cancernet .nci.nih.gov and the National Surgical Adjuvant Breast and Bowel Project (NSABP) can be accessed at http://www.nsabp.pitt.edu/ NSABP_Protocols.html

❖ Novel and Targeted Therapy

+ Targeted therapy extends from the DNA to include multiple features of the tumor cell. New targets include tyrosine kinase receptors such as epidermal growth factor receptor and HER-2, adhesion molecules, matrix proteins, and signal transduction molecules.

+ HER-2 gene that encodes the growth factor receptor HER-2 is amplified and HER-2 is overexpressed in 25%–30% of patients with breast cancer.

+ Trastuzumab is a recombinant monoclonal antibody against HER-2 and has shown significant activity and improved survival in patients with advanced breast cancer amplifying the HER-2 gene.[10]

+ Trastuzumab is being evaluated in the adjuvant setting. However, because cardiac toxicity has been observed in the trastuzumab/anthracycline combination, a sequential approach adding trastuzumab to anthracycline based chemotherapy strategy has been developed.[11,12]

+ Trastuzumab is being evaluated in Intergroup/ North Central Cancer Treatment Group in patients with HER-2 positive disease.

+ See Table 9-5.

❖ Hormonal Therapy in Primary Breast Cancer

+ Tamoxifen is a nonsteroidal compound that binds to estrogen receptors and has both estrogen antagonist and estrogen agonist properties. Drugs that exhibit dual activities are referred to as *selective estrogen receptor modulators* (SERMs).

❖ Tamoxifen Benefits

+ Preserves bone mineral density in postmenopausal women

+ Exerts favorable effect on blood lipid profiles

+ Anti-estrogen effects are mediated by competitive blockade of ER resulting in reduced transcription of estrogen-regulated genes. Results in blockade of cell cycle transit in G1 phase and inhibition of tumor growth.

TABLE 9-5
Targeted Therapy

Trastuzumab (Herceptin)

Mechanism of action	Recombinant humanized monoclonal anti-HER-2 antibody
	Targets extracellular domain of HER-2 growth factor receptor
	Inhibits signal transduction and cell proliferation
Indications/Use	Overexpression/amplification of HER-2/neu (c-erbB-2) metastatic breast cancer
Range of dosage	4 mg/kg IV loading dose over 90 minutes; then 2 mg/kg IV over 30 minutes weekly
Special precautions	During first infusion, mild to moderate chills and fever that usually abate with subsequent treatment
	Cardiotoxicity is a rare complication and may occur in patients previously treated with anthracyclines
Toxicity	Nausea, vomiting, and pain are infrequent side effects
	Other side effects include increased anemia, leukopenia, diarrhea, and infection

❖ NIH Consensus Development Statement on Adjuvant Hormonal Therapy[2]

+ Adjuvant hormonal therapy is recommended to women whose breast cancers express hormone receptor protein, regardless of age, menopausal status, involvement of axillary lymph nodes, or tumor size.

+ Five years of tamoxifen 20 mg per day is standard adjuvant hormone therapy.

+ Chemotherapy and tamoxifen combined improves survival in women with hormone receptor-positive tumors compared with tamoxifen alone.

+ Tamoxifen is associated with a slight increased risk of endometrial cancer and venous thrombosis but the potential benefits of tamoxifen outweigh risks for the majority of women.

+ Ovarian ablation is an alternative for select premenopausal women.

+ Tamoxifen combined with polychemotherapy further reduces the risk of disease recurrence and should be considered for premenopausal women.

❖ **Side Effects of Tamoxifen**

+ In general, tamoxifen is well tolerated.

+ Hot flashes occur in 50%–60% of women and is more common in premenopausal women.

+ Depression is an uncommon side effect but symptoms may be severe and may require either dose reduction, antidepressant medication, or discontinuation of tamoxifen.

+ Women with pre-existing cataracts taking tamoxifen may have a slightly increased risk of posterior subcapsular opacities but no vision-threatening ocular toxicity.

+ Thrombolic and hematologic toxicities occur more frequently when tamoxifen is combined with chemotherapy.

+ Severe thromboembolic events occur in less than 1% of patients.

+ Endometrial and other cancers (e.g., liver cancer) are most troublesome side effect of long-term tamoxifen.

+ See Table 9-6 for effects of tamoxifen.

❖ **Promising New Research Directions for Adjuvant Hormonal Therapy**

+ Risks and benefits of continuing tamoxifen longer than 5 years

TABLE 9-6
Acute and Adverse Effects of Tamoxifen

Acute and Transient Effects	*Serious Adverse Effects*
Gastrointestinal upset	Thromboembolic events
Symptoms of estrogen withdrawal	Elevated endometrial cancer risk
Hot flashes	Occular toxicity (retinopathy, cataracts)
Vaginal bleeding/discharge	
Menstrual irregularities	
Depression	

+ Value of combined hormonal therapy

+ Risks and benefits of new selective estrogen
  receptor modulators (SERM) and aromatase
  inhibitors and inactivators

SELECTED REFERENCES

1. Osborne, C. K., & Ravdin, P. M. (2000). Adjuvant
   systemic therapy of primary breast cancer. In J. R.
   Harris, M. Lippman, M. Morrow, & C. K. Osborne
   (Eds.), *Diseases of the breast*, (2nd ed., pp. 599–632).
   Philadelphia: Lippincott Williams & Wilkins.)

2. National Institutes of Health. NIH Consensus
   Development Conference Statement on Adjuvant
   Therapy for Breast Cancer, November 1–3, 2000.
   Available online at http://odp.od.nih.gov/consensus/
   cons/114/114_statement.htm

3. Perez, E. (2001). Doxorubicin and paclitaxel in the
   treatment of advanced breast cancer: Efficacy and
   cardiac considerations. *Cancer Investigation, 19,* 155–164.

4. Nabholtz, J-M., & Riva, A. (2001). Taxane/anthracycline combinations: Setting a new standard in breast cancer? *The Oncologist, 6*(suppl 3), 5–12.

5. Holmes, F. A., Walters, R. S., Theriault, R. L., et al. (1991). Phase II trial of TAXOL, an active drug in the treatment of metastatic breast cancer. *Journal of the National Cancer Institute, 83,* 1897–1905.

6. Nabholtz, J. M., Gelmon, K., Bontebal, M., et al. (1996). Multicenter, randomized, comparative study of two doses of paclitaxel in patients with metastatic breast cancer. *Journal of Clinical Oncology, 14,* 1858–1867.

7. CALGB9344, U.S. Food and Drug Administration (FDA) hearing, September, 1999.

8. Henderson, I. C., Berry, D., Demetri, C., et al. (1998). Improved disease-free survival (DFS) and overall survival (OS) from the addition of sequential paclitaxel (T), but not from the escalation of doxorubicin (A) dose level in the adjuvant chemotherapy of patients (PTS) with node-positive primary breast cancer (BC). *Proceedings of the American Society of Clinical Oncology, 17,* 101a.

9. Norton, L. (2001). Theoretical concepts and the emerging role of taxanes in adjuvant therapy. *The Oncologist, 6*(Suppl 3), 30–35.

10. Slamon, D., Goddphin, W., Jones, L. A., et al. (1989). Studies of the HER-2/neu proto-oncogene in human breast and ovarian cancer. *Science, 244,* 707–712.

11. Nabholtz, J., & Slamon, D. (2001). New adjuvant strategies for breast cancer: Meeting the challenge of

integrating chemotherapy and trastuzumab (Herceptin). *Seminars in Oncology, 118*(1 Suppl 3), 1–12.

12. Slamon, D., & Pegram, M. (2001). Rationale for trastuzumab (Herceptin) in adjuvant breast cancer trials. *Seminars in Oncology, 28*(1Suppl 3), 13–19.

10

Symptom Management of Acute Side Effects of Adjuvant Chemotherapy

❖ **Adjuvant Chemotherapy: Acute Side Effects**

+ Most women with primary breast cancer tolerate adjuvant chemotherapy very well.

+ Some modifications in normal lifestyle and routine are needed during treatment.

+ Patients are able to continue working.

❖ **Nursing Role in Management**

+ Educate the patient and family.

+ Provide emotional support for the patient and family.

+ Coordinate patient care.

+ Facilitate support groups.

+ Manage the side effects of treatment.

❖ **Acute and Expected Side Effects**

+ Grade 3 or 4 neutropenia

+ Alopecia or hair loss

+ Nausea and vomiting

+ Thromboembolic events

+ Weight gain

+ Mucositis

+ Fatigue

+ Arthralgia/myalgia

❖ **Neutropenia[1]**

+ Definition: Reduction in the number of circulating neutrophils of less than 1,000/μL

+ Neutropenia is the largest predictor of infection in patients with cancer.

+ Absolute neutrophil count (ANC) is calculated by the following formula: segmented neutrophils (%) + bands (%) × white blood cell count = ANC

+ Risk levels

   ANC >1,500/μL = normal risk

   ANC <1,000/μL = moderate risk

   ANC <500/μL = severe risk

   ANC <100/μL = extreme risk

+ Short-term neutropenia lasts less than a week.

+ Long-term neutropenia exceeds 1 to 2 weeks.

+ Risk factors include advancing age and concurrent or prior radiation therapy.

+ Chemotherapy agents used in breast cancer that increase risk of neutropenia: doxorubicin, cyclophosphamide, paclitaxel, methotrexate

+ Neutropenic episodes during chemotherapy are predictable, with the nadir (or lowest) WBC occurring 10 to 14 days after treatment, with full recovery 3 to 4 weeks after treatment.

+ Signs and symptoms

> *Fever with temperature higher than 38°C (100°F) or 100.4° in a 24-hour period, or temperature spike of 38.5°C or 101.3°F*

> *Pain and tenderness*

> *Change in character or color of urine, sputum, or stool*

> *Breaks in skin integrity*

> *Dysuria or frequency of urination*

> *Malaise, lethargy, myalgia*

> *In moderate to severe neutropenia, objective signs of infection are generally absent.*

+ Prevention of neutropenia

> *Hematopoietic growth factors decrease the severity of neutropenia.*

+ Management of neutropenia

   Prompt recognition and work-up for suspected area of infection

   Physical assessment, blood cultures, chest radiograph (CXR), and other studies as needed

   Antibiotic therapy

+ Patient self-care management

   Monitor temperature at least twice daily.

   Use steps to decrease colonization, such as dietary changes and avoidance of individuals with known or suspected infections.

   Practice good skin and self-care hygiene.

   Implement precautions to reduce risk of upper respiratory infection.

❖ **Hair Loss[2-4]**

+ While most discussions of hair loss focus on scalp hair, there is also loss of hair in the axilla, pubis, eyebrows, and eyelashes.

+ Degrees of hair loss

   Total hair loss occurs with doxorubicin.

   High potential for hair loss or alopecia occurs with cyclophosphamide and paclitaxel.

   Moderate potential for hair loss occurs with methotrexate and 5-fluorouracil (5-FU).

> *Hair thinning and moderate hair loss occurs with cyclophosphamide, methotrexate, and 5-fluorouracil (CMF).*

+ Hair loss typically begins around 2 to 3 weeks after first exposure to chemotherapy, with continued loss over 3 to 4 weeks.

+ Differences in the rate of hair loss can occur.

> *Hair loss with paclitaxel occurs around 2 to 3 weeks and may be sudden and cumulative.*

+ Common Toxicity Criteria of the National Cancer Institute provide a set of measures of commonly experienced side effects of clinical trials to help decrease the subjectivity of measurement (Table 10-1).

+ Prevention of hair loss

> *Scalp tourniquets and scalp hypothermia or cooling agents were used during the 1980s; widespread use of prevention techniques has declined.*

+ Focus on hair loss management has shifted to that of preparatory information.

TABLE 10-1
Common Toxicity Criteria of the National Cancer Institute

Grade 0	Grade 1	Grade 2	Grade 3	Grade 4
Normal	Mild hair loss	Pronounced hair loss	—	—

Help the patient anticipate hair loss and prepare for it.

Obtain a wig to fit normal hair color and style prior to beginning chemotherapy.

Suggest turbans and hats to protect the scalp during chemotherapy.

Access the services of the American Cancer Society (ACS) "Look Good . . . Feel Better" Program for community information and support.

Suggest cutting the hair to a manageable style before chemotherapy begins.

Use mild shampoo and conditioner.

Avoid electric curlers and curling irons.

Avoid excessive hair brushing.

When hair loss begins, it may occur in a rapid manner, or the hair may thin over time.

Scalp and skin around the ears may become itchy and dry, requiring mild soap and soothing emollients or lotions.

✦ Hair loss is temporary, and regrowth may be seen 3 months after completion of chemotherapy.

New hair color may differ from the original color.

Hair texture also may differ from that of the original hair (may be softer and finer).

❖ Nausea and Vomiting[5,6]

+ Doxorubicin, epirubicin, cyclophosphamide (oral and intravenous), fluorouracil, and paclitaxel doses used in breast cancer treatment are considered moderate to moderately high emetogenic agents.

+ Patient characteristics that place them at risk for nausea and vomiting include female gender, younger age, and a history of motion sickness or hyperemesis in pregnancy.

+ Patients at lower risk for nausea and vomiting are those with a history of chronic, daily, high alcohol intake.

+ The NCI grading criteria for nausea and vomiting is listed on Table 10-2.

+ Mechanisms of nausea and vomiting

TABLE 10-2
Common Toxicity Criteria for Nausea and Vomiting

	Grade 0	Grade 1	Grade 2	Grade 3	Grade 4
Nausea	None	Able to eat reasonable intake	Intake significantly decreased but can eat	No significant intake	>10 episodes in 24, hours requiring parenteral support
Vomiting	None	One episode in 24 hours	2–5 episodes in 24 hours	6–10 episodes in 24 hours	

TABLE 10-3

Classification of Nausea and Vomiting

Acute	Delayed	Anticipatory	Refractory
Occurs within 24 hours of chemotherapy	Occurs after 24 hours after chemotherapy and lasts up to 5 days	Occurs before chemotherapy and is related to poor nausea and vomiting control during prior treatment	Unresponsive to anti-emetic therapy

+ Classification of nausea and vomiting are in Table 10-3

   Central stimulation of the brain's vomiting center and chemoreceptor trigger zone (CTZ)

   Peripheral stimulation of enterochromaffin cells in the gastrointestinal (GI) tract

❖ **Classification of Antiemetics[7]**

   + 5-HT$_3$ receptor antagonists

   + Dopamine antagonists

   + Corticosteroids

   + Benzodiazepines

      Used for anticipatory nausea and vomiting and anxiety

❖ **Serotonin Antagonists**

   + With the advent and use of 5-HT$_3$ receptor

serotonin antagonists (e.g., ondansetron, granisetron, dolasetron), acute nausea and vomiting are well controlled.

+ Granisetron, ondansetron, and dolasetron provide equivalent protection for moderately to highly emetogenic drugs.

+ $5\text{-}HT_3$ receptor antagonists bind to serotonin receptors on the afferent vagus and splanchnic nerves in the GI tract and CTZ for about 24 hours.

+ These agents work within the vomiting center of the brain and on the enterochromaffin cells in the gut.

+ These agents are first-line therapy for moderately to highly emetogenic chemotherapy.

+ Improved anti-emetic response when ondansetron is used in combination with dexamethasone 20 mg

+ Second-line antiemetic therapy for patients with problematic side effects from other antiemetics

+ These agents are not as effective for control of delayed nausea and vomiting.

Side effects include headache, constipation, lightheadedness, and sedation.

❖ **Dopamine Antagonists**

+ Metoclopramide, phenothiazines, and

butyrophenones bind to dopamine receptors and block impulses from the vomiting center

+ These agents are used to treat nausea and vomiting from low to moderate emetogenic chemotherapy, and delayed nausea and vomiting.

+ Major disadvantage is that these agents cause extrapyramidal reactions, with the most common symptom called *akathisia* ("dancing legs").

+ Metoclopramide is used for acute and delayed nausea and vomiting.

+ Phenothiazines are used for acute nausea and vomiting from mildly emetogenic chemotherapy and for delayed and persistent nausea and vomiting.

+ Butyrophenones are dopamine antagonists similar to phenothiazines.

❖ **Corticosteroids**

+ Mechanism of action as an antiemetic is unknown, but corticosteroids have both central and peripheral effects.

   May decrease capillary permeability of CNS

+ Increase anti-emetic effect of 5-HT$_3$ by 20%

+ Useful for delayed nausea and vomiting

+ Insomnia is a bothersome side effect.

❖ **Benzodiazepines**

+ Modest antiemetic effect, and are thus combined with other antiemetics

+ Mechanism of antiemetic action is unknown.

+ Lorazepam decreases anxiety and agitation and may alter the perception of nausea and vomiting.

+ Lorazepam may be used to minimize anticipatory nausea and vomiting.

❖ **Nonpharmacologic Interventions**

+ Behavioral interventions

   Guided imagery, hypnosis, relaxation techniques, massage therapy, music therapy, and biofeedback

   Helpful in managing anticipatory nausea and vomiting

+ Acupressure

❖ **Nutritional Modification**

+ Change to a bland diet or foods that do not have offensive odor or spicy taste

+ Cold or room-temperature foods

+ Clear liquids, carbonated beverages, and soda crackers

+ Avoidance of high-fat foods, which can delay gastric emptying

❖ Thromboembolic Events

+ More common when chemotherapy is combined with tamoxifen

+ Lethal toxicity occurs more frequently in postmenopausal women.

❖ Stomatitis/Mucositis[8]

+ *Stomatitis and mucositis* is a general term referring to inflammation and ulceration of the oral mucosa (Table 10-4).

+ Oral mucosa is vulnerable to the effects of chemotherapy because the cells live for about 5 days and there is a rapid turnover of the epithelial lining every 7 to 14 days

+ Chemotherapy has a direct and indirect stomatoxic effect, and stomatitis is usually associated with chemotherapy.

TABLE 10-4

National Cancer Institute Common Toxicity Grading Criteria for Stomatitis

Grade 0	Grade 1	Grade 2	Grade 3	Grade 4
None	Painless ulcers, erythema, or mild soreness	Painful erythema, edema, or ulcers but can eat	Painful erythema, edema, or ulcers, and cannot eat	Requires parenteral or enteral support

+ A chemotherapy agent associated with high degree of stomatitis is fluorouracil.

+ Other chemotherapy agents include doxorubicin and methotrexate.

+ Patients at higher risk for stomatitis/neurositis

  Poor oral hygiene

  Presence of dental caries

  Chronic alcohol use

+ Stomatitis is predictable and occurs within 2 to 5 days after treatment and can persist up to 14 days.

+ Prevention strategies[9]

  Primary goal is prevention of stomatitis.

  Implement a good oral hygiene program and maintain a good nutritional state.

  Agents used for oral care are cleansing agents (e.g., normal saline, hydrogen peroxide rinses) and lubricating agents (e.g., emollients).

+ Management of mild to moderate stomatitis

  Assess oral cavity.

  Promote oral hygiene.

  Use mouth rinses.

  Change to a soft, high-calorie diet.

  Culture any suspicious oral lesions.

Continue with cleansing agents and lubricating agents.

Use topical anesthetics (e.g., benzocaine, Zilactin)

✦ Management of severe stomatitis

Warm saline rinses

Antifungal/antibacterial oral suspension

Oxidizing agents

Culture lesion and monitor for secondary oral infections

Use topical/systemic analgesics

Maintain hydration

❖ **Weight Gain**

✦ Incidence of weight gain varies between 50% and 90%.

✦ Weight gain greater than 10% of body weight, up to 22 pounds

✦ Mechanism of weight gain may be related to sarcopenic obesity.

✦ May last up to 2 years post-treatment

✦ Interventions

Anticipatory guidance

Documentation of weight

Nutritional counseling

> *Exercise (e.g., self-paced walking programs, fitness exercises)*

❖ Cancer-Related Fatigue[10]

+ Reader is referred to Chapter 15 for further discussion of cancer-related fatigue (CRF)

+ Most frequently reported side effect of treatment

+ Includes physical sensations of tiredness, mental slowness, and lack of emotional resilience[11]

+ Intensity and patterns fluctuate, based on treatment.

+ Physiologic mechanisms of fatigue are unknown.

+ Assessment of CRF

> *Modeled on similar approach to pain assessment, using 0 to 10 scale, on which 0 is no fatigue and 10 is the most fatigue possible.*

+ Management of CRF

> *Prepare patients for its occurrence.*

> *Provide instructions about balance of energy conservation and appropriate exercise.*

> *Assist patients in prioritizing activities that differentiate essential from nonessential tasks.*

> *Promote a balance between sleep and rest—patients who are fatigued may also experience accompanying symptom clusters of sleep disruption and mood disturbance.*

Evaluate the effectiveness of the interventions.

+ Exercise as an intervention

    Research suggests that women receiving adjuvant chemotherapy benefit from either supervised or a self-administered walking exercise program.

❖ **Arthralgia/Myalgia[11]**

+ Arthralgia is joint pain.

+ Myalgia is diffuse muscle pain.

+ Symptoms are dose-related.

    Paclitaxel at doses less than 170 mg/m² causes mild discomfort.

    Paclitaxel at doses greater than 200 mg/m² is associated with more severe discomfort and pain.

    Overlapping side effects of other chemotherapy include fatigue, malaise, decreased appetite, and lack of energy.

+ Symptom management (Table 10-5)

    Perform a careful assessment to identify risk factors.

    Inform patients as to what to expect, what can be prevented, and to whom to report side effects, timeline of toxicity.

    Treatment approaches

    Antihistamines, corticosteroids, NSAIDs, opiates

    Warm bath, relaxation techniques, massage therapy

TABLE 10-5

National Cancer Institute Common Toxicity Grading Criteria for Arthralgia and Myalgia

Grade 0	Grade 1	Grade 2	Grade 3	Grade 4
None	Mild pain: not interfering with function	Moderate pain: pain or analgesics interfering with function but not interfering with activities of daily living	Severe pain: pain or analgesics severely interfering with activities of daily living	Disabling

REFERENCES

1. Wujcik, D. (1999). Infection. In C. H. Yarbro, M. H. Frogge, & M. Goodman (Eds.), *Cancer symptom management* (2nd ed., pp. 307–321). Sudbury, MA: Jones and Bartlett.

2. Reeves, D. (1999). Alopecia. In C. H. Yarbro, M. H. Frogge, & M. Goodman (Eds.), *Cancer symptom management* (2nd ed., pp. 275–284). Sudbury, MA: Jones and Bartlett.

3. Williams, J., Wood, C. L., & Cunningham-Warburton, P. (1999). A narrative study of chemotherapy-induced alopecia. *Oncology Nursing Forum, 26*, 1463–1468.

4. Pickard-Holley, S. (1995). The symptom experience of alopecia. *Seminars in Oncology Nursing, 11*, 235–238.

5. Wickham, R. (1999). Nausea and vomiting. In C. H.

Yarbro, M. H. Frogge, & M. Goodman (Eds.), *Cancer symptom management* (2nd ed., pp. 228–263). Sudbury, MA: Jones and Bartlett.

6. Hesketh, P. (1999). Defining the emetogenicity of cancer chemotherapy regimens: Relevance to clinical practice. *Oncologist, 4,* 191–196.

7. Wilkes, G., Ingwersen, K., & Barton-Burke, M. (2000). Nausea and vomiting. In *Oncology nursing drug handbook* (pp. 418–447). Sudbury, MA: Jones and Bartlett.

8. Beck, S. Mucositis. (1999). In C. H. Yarbro, M. H. Frogge, & M. Goodman (Eds.), *Cancer symptom management* (2nd ed., pp. 328–343). Sudbury, MA: Jones and Bartlett.

9. Steel, R. (1999). *Handbook of cancer chemotherapy* (5th ed.). Philadelphia: Lippincott Williams and Wilkins.

10. Winningham, M. (1999). Fatigue. In C. H. Yarbro, M. H. Frogge, & M. Goodman (Eds.), *Cancer symptom management* (2nd ed., pp. 58–76). Sudbury, MA: Jones and Bartlett.

11. Martin, V. (2000). Arthralgias and myalgias. In C. H. Yarbro, M. H. Frogge, & M. Goodman (Eds.), *Cancer symptom management* (2nd ed., pp. 35–44). Sudbury, MA: Jones and Bartlett.

PART III

Treatment of Recurrent and Metastatic Breast Cancer

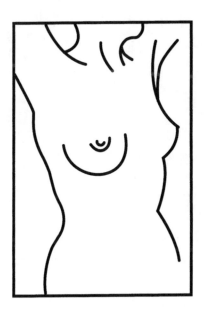

11

Local Treatment of Recurrent and Metastatic Disease

- *Local recurrence* is defined as the reappearance of cancer in the ipsilateral breast, chest wall, or skin overlying the chest wall after initial treatment.

- *Regional recurrence* is defined as the appearance of tumor involving the ipsilateral axillary lymph nodes, supraclavicular lymph nodes, infraclavicular lymph nodes, and internal mammary lymph nodes.

- Local recurrence may occur after either mastectomy or breast-conserving surgery (BCS) and radiation therapy (XRT).

❖ Local Recurrence after Mastectomy[1]

- Local recurrence often presents as one or more asymptomatic nodules in or under the skin of the chest wall.

+ Nodules are located in or near the mastectomy scar or skin graft, and after reconstruction with a myocutaneous flap.

+ Recurrence may look like an erythematous, pruritic skin rash.

+ Eighty percent to 90% of local recurrences are evident within 5 years after mastectomy.

+ Twenty-five percent to 33% of patients with local or regional recurrence have distant metastasis before local recurrence is found.

+ About 25% of patients develop simultaneous local and distant metastasis within a few months after local recurrence.

+ Unfortunately, nearly all patients with local recurrence after mastectomy develop distant metastasis.

❖ **Treatment of Local Recurrence after Mastectomy**

+ XRT is generally given to the chest wall and supraclavicular nodes.

> With a higher dose of radiation to a large chest wall field and nodal irradiation, the higher is the likelihood of local control.

> Recurrence in a mastectomy scar may be more difficult to control, compared with other chest wall recurrence.

> *Patients who have local failure after mastectomy and reconstruction have control rates and outcomes similar to other patients without reconstruction.*

> *Radiation to the internal mammary nodes requires a larger volume of lung and heart (for left-sided lesions) in the treatment field, which may increase patient morbidity, particularly after prior doxorubicin-based adjuvant therapy.*

> *Axillary radiation is not generally done unless there is clinical involvement or minimal dissection.*

✦ Radiation treatment consists of either photon radiation or mixed photon-electron beam radiation.

> *45 to 50 Gy, using photons delivered in 1.8- to 2.0-Gy fractions five times a week to chest wall*

> *10- to 20-Gy boost with photons or electrons to areas of gross disease and biopsy*

> *Total radiation dose of 60 Gy*

✦ Side effects and complications

> *Acute side effects include a brisk skin redness and possible desquamation.*

> *Complications include telangiectasia and mild subcutaneous fibrosis.*

> *Serious complications, such as radiation pneumonitis, soft-tissue necrosis, bone necrosis, and neuropathy, are rare.*

Concurrent administration of chemotherapy may increase the risk of pneumonitis, pericarditis, and brachial plexopathy.

❖ **Treatment of Local Recurrence after Breast-Conserving Surgery and Radiation Therapy (BCS + XRT)**

+ About 50% of local recurrence after BCS and XRT are detected by mammography.

+ Physical and radiologic characteristics of recurrent tumors are similar to those of initial tumors.

+ Physical examination shows mild thickening without a mass; in some patients, recurrence may produce only mild thickening or retraction at the biopsy site.

+ Prognosis after recurrence in BCS + XRT is better than local recurrence after mastectomy.

+ Treatment with salvage mastectomy is the standard therapy.

Mastectomy has a 5-year, relapse-free survival rate of about 60% to 75%.

+ Postoperative complications include delayed wound healing and infection.

+ Patients desiring immediate reconstruction may have a higher risk of delayed wound healing and a variable cosmetic result because of prior XRT.

❖ Most Common Sites of Metastatic Breast Cancer

- ✦ Bone
- ✦ Epidural spinal cord
- ✦ Brain

❖ Bone Metastases[2]

- ✦ Most frequent site of metastasis, with about 90% of patients with metastatic disease having bone metastases

- ✦ Lesions may be osteolytic, osteoblastic, mixed osteolytic-osteoblastic, and osteoporotic, leading to pathologic fractures of weight-bearing bones.

- ✦ Bone metastases occur in trabecular bone and cortical bones.

- ✦ Most common involved sites include pelvis, lumbar spine, thoracic spine, ribs, long bones, skull, and cervical spine.

- ✦ Bone metastasis is associated with bone loss and excess excretion of calcium.

- ✦ Symptoms of pain and disability, causing major problems in quality of life

- ✦ Work-up for bone metastases

    Physical examination, bone scan, and plain films

    Computed tomography (CT) and magnetic resonance imaging (MRI) also may be used in the evaluation.

❖ **Treatment of Bone Metastasis with Radiation Therapy**

✦ XRT is used for pain relief and prevention of impending pathologic fracture.

✦ Hemibody radiation has been used when there are multiple bony lesions in the spine.

✦ Side effects of radiation therapy for bone metastasis

Skin erythema in treatment field

Mild to moderate fatigue

✦ Strontium-89, a radioactive isotope, may be given by intravenous injection for relief of bone pain.

Preferentially taken up at sites of active bone tumor, with higher uptake in metastatic disease

Useful for patients with diffuse bony metastasis

Hematologic toxicity is dose-limiting toxicity.

✦ 153-Ethylenediaminetetramethylenephosphonate (153-EDTMP), a second bone-seeking radioactive agent is also available with more limited efficacy studies of its use.

✦ Pain management for bone metastasis

Patients require an effective pain control regimen during XRT.

Combination of opioid and nonopioid (NSAID) helps relieve pain during XRT.

Bisphosphonates help to reduce pain.

❖ Treatment of Bone Metastasis with Bisphosphonates

+ Bisphosphonates are analogues of pyrophosphate and have been shown to inhibit osteoclast-mediated bone destruction.

+ Although the mechanism of action is not known, they are thought to preferentially localize at sites of active bone remodeling and osteolysis.

+ These agents also inhibit malignant bone disease and osteoporosis due to estrogen deficiency.

+ American Society of Clinical Oncology Guidelines established the role of bisphosphonates in the treatment of breast cancer[3]; the guidelines are available at http://guideline@asco.org

> *Benefit of bisphosphonates is reduction in skeletal complications, such as pathologic fracture, surgery for fracture or impending fracture, XRT, spinal cord compression, and hypercalcemia.*

> *Bisphosphonates provide a supportive but not life-prolonging benefit in patients with bone metastases.*

> *Pamidronate, 90 mg intravenously (IV), infused over 3 to 4 hours is recommended for patients with imaging evidence of lytic destruction of bone who are on concurrent hormonal therapy or chemotherapy.*

> *Once bisphosphonate therapy is started, it should be continued until there is evidence of a substantial decline in the patient's general performance status.*
>
> *Patients with an abnormal bone scan without bony destruction or localized pain are not recommended to start bisphosphonates.*
>
> *Bisphosphonates for patients at high risk for bone metastasis at any stage of non–bone disease should be evaluated in a clinical trial.*
>
> *Oral bisphosphonates can be used for preservation of bone density in premenopausal women with treatment-related menopause.*
>
> *Current standard of care using local XRT and pain management should not be displaced by bisphosphonates.*

+ Zoledronate is a newer bisphosphonate agent.

> *The effect of zoledronate on the need for XRT and change in pain was recently evaluated.*
>
> *Four milligrams IV over 5 minutes was demonstrated as effective as pamidronate IV.*
>
> *Shorter infusion time may offer time-saving advantage.*

❖ **Epidural Metastases[4]**

+ Epidural spinal cord compression is considered an oncologic emergency.

+ Predictors of spinal cord compression include known bone metastases to the spine of at least 2 years, metastatic disease at initial diagnosis, and weakness.[5]

+ Spinal cord damage is due to direct compression of the spinal cord by tumor.

+ Breast cancer accounts for 7% to 32% of all cases of spinal cord compression.

+ Signs and symptoms

    Pain is the most common initial symptom and precedes other symptoms by several weeks.

    Pain is local, radicular, and referred, and the type of pain is further described in Table 11-1.

    Pain worsens when patients are lying down and when patients use stretch maneuvers such as neck flexion.

    Myelopathy symptoms such as limb weakness, numbness, and paresthesias, and sphincter disturbance may occur.

    Prognosis with spinal cord compression is related to clinical deficits at the time of presentation

+ If left untreated, epidural spinal cord compression (ESCC) complications include paraplegia or quadriplegia.

+ Work-up includes plain spine films, radionuclide bone scan, CT of the spine, and MRI.

Table 11-1

Types of Pain Related to Spinal Cord Compression

Type of Pain	Description of Pain
Local	Described as a constant ache Occurs in nearly all patients
Radicular	Described as a shooting pain Caused by involvement of nerve roots by the tumor More common in cervical and lumbosacral lesions
Referred	Occurs at a site distant from the lesion Pain does not radiate Lesions in the lower thoracic and lumbar spine may be referred to iliac crests or sacroiliac joints Lesions in low cervical and high thoracic regions may be referred to interscapular region or shoulders

❖ Treatment of Epidural Spinal Cord Compression (SCC)

✦ Corticosteroids

Routinely used to reduce pain and stabilize neurologic deficits

Usually, a larger bolus dose of dexamethasone, followed by a tapering dose over several weeks while patient receives definitive therapy, is indicated.

✦ XRT

Emergency treatment with XRT should be started on an urgent basis.

Recommended first-line treatment, using a dose up to 30 Gy delivered in 3-Gy fractions to the targeted area in spine

✦ Surgery

May be used in selected situations in which patients' disease progresses or relapses with XRT

Decompressive laminectomy has very limited effectiveness.

❖ **Management of Treatment Side Effects from Radiation Therapy**

✦ General skin-care measures during XRT

✦ XRT for SCC may result in mild to moderate local side effects, depending on the bodily structures in the path of the radiation beam.

✦ XRT to the cervical spine may cause dysphagia.

Nutritional measures, such as increasing liquids and instituting a soft diet

Local anesthetic for pain

❖ **Brain Metastases[6]**

✦ Brain metastases is the most common neurologic complication in breast cancer, occurring in about 15% of patients.

✦ Majority of patients are treated with palliative external beam whole-brain XRT, with relief of symptoms occurring in about 45% of patients.

+ Median time from diagnosis to CNS metastases is about 33 months, with median survival after treatment of about 4 months.[7]

+ Patients with singular brain metastasis with postoperative radiation have better survival, compared with patients with multiple brain metastases and meningeal spread.

+ Hematogenous spread is the most common mechanism of brain metastases.

+ Brain metastases are more likely to occur in premenopausal women with aggressive and disseminated disease.

+ Development of brain metastases is delayed in patients who received adjuvant chemotherapy or hormonal therapy, but overall survival is not affected.

+ Signs and symptoms

 Signs and symptoms are variable, with the majority of patients presenting with progressive neurologic deficits, cognitive dysfunction, and seizure.

 Clinical manifestations include headache, altered mental status, hemiparesis, papilledema, and ataxia.

 Cognitive dysfunction includes memory problems and mood or personality changes.

+ Work-up

    CT scan detects the majority of brain metastases.

    Contrast-enhanced MRI is more sensitive than CT.

❖ **Symptomatic Treatment of Brain Metastases**

+ Corticosteroids with dexamethasone are routinely used to reduce symptomatic edema.

    Usual starting dose is 10 mg/day, followed by 4 mg qid.

    Patients have symptomatic relief within a few days after starting treatment.

    Side effects of corticosteroids include weight gain, myopathy, fluid retention, hyperglycemia, insomnia, gastritis, and immunosuppression.

+ Anticonvulsant therapy in patients presenting with seizures

    Routine anticonvulsant therapy in patients who have not experienced seizure is not indicated.

    The side effect of drug rashes is not uncommon.

    Very small percentage of patients develop Stevens-Johnson syndrome while on anticonvulsant therapy.

❖ **Definitive Treatment of Brain Metastases**

+ Treatment is delivered on an emergency basis.

+ Goals of definitive treatment are symptomatic relief of symptoms and improvement of local control of disease.

+ XRT to whole brain on an emergency basis and surgery are the major treatments for brain metastases.

❖ **Radiation Therapy**

+ XRT is the standard treatment of brain metastases and is also effective in palliating neurologic symptoms.

+ Up to 90% high response to radiation in decreasing neurologic symptoms.

+ Dose fractionation schedules vary from 30 Gy in 2 weeks to 40 Gy in 4 weeks

+ In general, patients who are treated in the shortest amount of time with larger radiation treatment fractions tend to respond more quickly.

+ Duration of response is equivalent with both fractionation schedules.

+ Late complications of XRT may include leukoencephalopathy, neurocognitive deterioration, and dementia.

+ Stereotactic radiosurgery is a technique that delivers a high single dose of radiation to a specific treatment volume and has been used for treatment of brain metastases.

Stereotactic radiosurgery can be done using high-energy x-rays from a linear accelerator or with gamma rays from a gamma knife.

◆ Side effects of XRT to whole brain[8]

Complete but temporary hair loss within a few weeks of start of XRT, with hair regrowth after treatment ends

Scalp dryness and itchiness

Skin erythema (especially in forehead and periauricular areas)

Fatigue

Potential for a transient increase in neurologic symptoms at start of XRT

◆ General skin-care guidelines

Use of a mild shampoo, such as baby shampoo, with gentle rinsing and towel drying

Avoidance of hair dryers, curling irons, and harsh chemicals (such as those used for dyeing and perming)

Patient teaching should include information regarding wigs, scarves, and protection of the scalp from summer sun or winter cold.

◆ Patient safety at home

Assess degree of cognitive impairment and need for home safety.

Monitor taper of steroids at the end of the treatment course.

Provide emotional support to patient and family.

❖ **Surgery for Brain Metastases**

✦ Used for treatment of single brain metastases that may be surgically resectable, which may be followed by stereotactic radiosurgery

✦ Used for treatment of multiple brain metastases with large symptomatic lesions, followed by whole-brain radiation

REFERENCES

1. Recht, A., Come, S., Troyan, S., & Sadowsky, N. Local-regional recurrence after mastectomy or breast-conserving therapy. (2000). In J. R. Harris, M. Lippman, M. Morrow, C. K. Osborne (Eds.), *Diseases of the breast* (2nd ed., pp. 731–748). Philadelphia: Lippincott Williams and Wilkins.

2. Theriault, R. (2000). Medical treatment of bone metastases. In J. R. Harris, M. Lippman, M. Morrow, C. K. Osborne (Eds.), *Diseases of the breast* (2nd ed., pp. 921–929). Philadelphia: Lippincott Williams and Wilkins.

3. Hillner, B., Ingle, J., Berrenson, J., et al. (2000). American Society of Clinical Oncology guideline on the role of bisphosphonates in breast cancer. American Society of

Clinical Oncology Bisphosphonates Expert Panel. *Journal of Clinical Oncology, 18,* 1378–1391.

4. McColl, C., & Freilich, R. (2000). Epidural metastases. In J. R. Harris, M. Lippman, M. Morrow, C. K. Osborne (Eds.), *Diseases of the breast* (2nd ed., pp. 855–865). Philadelphia: Lippincott Williams and Wilkins.

5. Lu, C., Stomper, P., Drislane, F., et al. (1998). Suspected spinal cord compression in breast cancer patients: A multidisciplinary risk assessment. *Breast Cancer Research and Treatment, 51,* 121–131.

6. Wen, P., & Shafman, T. (2000). Brain metastasis. In J. R. Harris, M. Lippman, M. Morrow, C. K. Osborne (Eds.), *Diseases of the breast* (2nd ed., pp. 841–853). Philadelphia: Lippincott Williams and Wilkins.

7. Fokstuen, T., Wilking, N., Rutqvist, L., et. al. (2000). Radiation therapy in the management of brain metastases from breast cancer. *Breast Cancer Research and Treatment, 62,* 211–216.

8. Bucholtz, J. (1997). Central nervous system tumors. In K. H. Dow, J. D. Bucholtz, R. Iwamoto, V. Fieler, & L. Hilderley (Eds.), *Nursing care in radiation oncology* (2nd ed., pp. 136–151). Philadelphia: WB Saunders.

12

Systemic Therapy and Targeted Therapy in Recurrent and Metastatic Disease[1]

✦ About 30% of patients develop metastases. Treatment for recurrent and metastatic disease differs from treatment for with early-stage disease. Women with metastatic disease are not cured by treatment. Rather, the goal of treatment is aimed at management of symptom, maintenance of quality of life, and potentially prolongation of survival.

> With systemic chemotherapy for recurrent and advanced disease, about 5% to 10% of patients may survive at least five years and 2% to 5% of patients become long-term survivors.

> Mean survival of patients is 18 to 24 months with a range of several months to several years.

Assessment of risk and benefit of treatment modalities on quality of life must be reviewed with patients prior to start of treatment.

1. Some patients are willing to accept a high degree of toxicity for even small survival benefits.

2. Other patients prefer minimal toxicity with some degree of symptom palliation.

Establish diagnosis of metastatic disease

1. Histologic diagnosis of suspicious lesions is indicated to determine predictive factors and selecting targeted therapy (e.g., patients with erb-b^2 positive tumors benefit from additional therapy).

Favorable prognostic indicators

1. Time interval between primary diagnosis and relapse with longer time interval of more than 5 years after treatment

2. Number and sites of metastatic disease with isolated sites of recurrence in the bone versus organ involvement

3. Visceral involvement is a poor prognostic indicator in metastasis.

There are two classes of therapeutic options: local or systemic. The reader is referred to Chapter 11 for further discussion of local treatment of recurrence and metastasis.

Systemic therapy includes chemotherapy, targeted or novel therapy, or endocrine therapy.

Selection of local, systemic therapy, targeted therapy, or combination of therapies is individualized

Figure 12-1 and Figure 12-2 show a decision algorithm for patients with metastatic breast cancer.[1]

FIGURE 12-1

Endocrine therapy for recurrent and metastatic breast cancer.

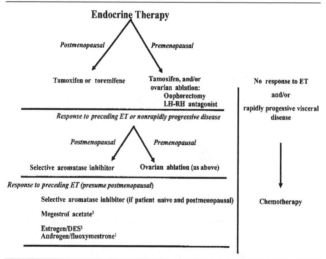

Source: Reprinted with permission from Ellis, M., Hayes, D., & Lippman, M. Treatment of metastatic breast cancer. In: J. R. Harris, M. Lippman, M. Morrow, C. K. Osborne (Eds.), *Diseases of the breast* (2nd ed., p. 756). Philadelphia: Lippincott Williams & Wilkins.

FIGURE 12-2
Chemotherapy for the treatment of recurrent and metastatic breast cancer

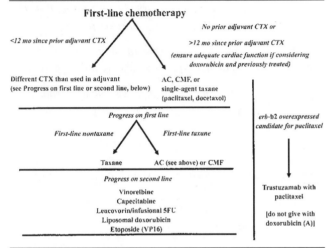

Source: Reprinted with permission from Ellis, M., Hayes, D., & Lippman, M. Treatment of metastatic breast cancer. In: J. R. Harris, M. Lippman, M. Morrow, C. K. Osborne (Eds.), *Diseases of the breast* (2nd ed., p. 757). Philadelphia: Lippincott Williams & Wilkins.

❖ Indications for Chemotherapy

- ✦ Patients with multiple metastatic sites and/or visceral disease are candidates for chemotherapy.

- ✦ Patients who are chemotherapy naïve have a higher likelihood of benefiting from chemotherapy.

- ✦ Patients with poorer response to chemotherapy

    Progression of disease while on prior chemotherapy

> *Recurrence within 12 months after completing adjuvant chemotherapy*
>
> *Poor performance status*
>
> *Increased number of metastatic sites including visceral involvement*

❖ **Selection of Chemotherapy in Metastatic Breast Cancer[1]**

+ Selection of type of chemotherapy and targeted therapy is based on individual patient factors.

+ Guidelines for treatment of metastatic breast cancer have been developed by the National Comprehensive Cancer Network (NCCN) in conjunction with the American Cancer Society and can be accessed at: http://www.nccn.org/ patient_guidelines/breast_cancer/breast/ 1_introduction.htm

+ First-line chemotherapy

> *When patients recur less than 12 months after initial chemotherapy, a chemotherapy regimen other than the chemotherapy used in the adjuvant setting is selected.*
>
> *When patients have not had prior adjuvant chemotherapy or more than 12 months has elapsed since prior adjuvant chemotherapy, combination AC, CMF, FAC/CAF with a taxane (i.e., paclitaxel or docetaxel)[2]*
>
> *Patients with HER2 (erbB2) overexpression are candidates for trastuzumab with paclitaxel.*

> *Several chemotherapy combinations are being evaluated as first-line treatment for metastatic breast cancer and include epidoxorubicin and docetaxel.[3]*

+ Second-line chemotherapy

> *When patients have progression of disease without prior taxane therapy, taxane may be indicated.*

> *When patients have had progression of disease with taxane, then AC or CMF may be indicated.*

> *Other chemotherapy agents used in metastatic disease that have different mechanisms of antitumor activity and toxicity profiles include gemcitabine, vinorelbine, capecitabine, leucovorin/infusional 5-FU, liposomal doxorubicin, and etoposide (VP16).[4,5,6,7,8]*

+ In addition to the chemotherapy drugs identified in Chapter 9, the agents in Table 12-1 are also used in the treatment of metastatic disease.

❖ **Targeted and Novel Therapy[12]**

+ Amplification and overexpression of protooncogene HER-2 or c-erb-b[2] is used to select patients for targeted trastuzumab therapy in metastatic disease.

> *C-erb-b[2] encodes a 185 kD transmembrane glycoprotein with tyrosine kinase activity that functions as a growth factor receptor.*

TABLE 12-1
Chemotherapy Used in Metastatic Breast Cancer[9,10,11]

Capecitabine (Xeloda)

Mechanism of action	Orally administered prodrug that converts to fluorouracil intracellularly
Indications/Use	Metastatic breast cancer resistant to anthracyclines and paclitaxel or cancer resistant to paclitaxel for whom further anthracycline therapy is not indicated
Range of dosage	2,500 mg/m² PO in two divided doses with food for 14 days; follow with 1 week rest; given as 3-week cycle
Special precautions	Diarrhea may be more severe in elderly patients
Toxicity	Diarrhea may be severe Hand and foot syndrome Dermatitis Grade 3–4 hematologic toxicity (neutropenia and thrombocytopenia) Nausea and vomiting: common Fatigue Anorexia and abdominal pain less common

Gemcitabine (Gemzar, difluorodeoxycitidine)

Mechanism of action	Antimetabolite Nucleoside analog inhibits ribonucleotide reductase and competes with deoxycytidine triphosphate for incorporation into DNA
Range of dosage	800–1,250 mg/m² IV on days 1, 8, and 15 of 28-day cycle
Special precautions	Irritant Administration: IV over 30 minutes up to 4 hours diluted in 100–200 cc of saline If >2,500 mg/m², dilute in 1,000 ml and infuse over 4 hours or longer Toxicity increased with longer infusion time

(continued)

TABLE 12-1
Chemotherapy Used in Metastatic Breast Cancer (*continued*)

Toxicity	Myelosuppression: common; dose-limiting
	Nausea and vomiting: common, not severe
	Diarrhea: occasional
	Constipation
	Rash, fever, flu-like symptoms with first dose
	Alopecia
	Increase in liver function tests

Vinorelbine (Navelbine)

Mechanism of action	Semi-synthetic vinca alkaloid
	Inhibits tubulin polymerization, inhibits mitosis
Indications/Use	Metastatic breast cancer
Range of dosage	30 mg/m² IV as rapid infusion weekly when used as a single agent
	20–25 mg/m² IV as rapid infusion in various schedules when used with other drugs
Special precautions	Vesicant
	Administer: IV in NS or D5W over 5–8 minutes with IV fluids running wide open; then flush with 200–300 ml of fluids
Toxicity	Myelosuppression: dose-limiting; nadir 7–10 days
	Nausea and vomiting: common; mild to moderate
	Neurotoxicity: less common than seen with vincristine
	Constipation, occasional paresthesia, tumor and jaw pain
	Alopecia: occasional
	Allergic reaction: chest pain, dyspnea, wheezing during administration; may premedicate with corticosteroids
	Be alert for chest pain in patients with tumor in chest or history of cardiovascular disease

> *Amplified or over-expressed HER-2/neu occurs in 25% to 30% of human breast cancer and is associated with rapid proliferation, growth, and metastasis.*

> *Trastuzumab is an anti-HER-2 monoclonal antibody indicated in patients with metastatic breast cancer with overexpression of HER-2, for first-line therapy with paclitaxel,[13] and as monotherapy in second-line and third-line treatment.*

> *The addition of trastuzumab to first-line chemotherapy in metastatic breast cancer is associated with a higher rate and duration of response and longer survival.[7]*

> *Trastuzumab can result in the development of ventricular dysfunction and congestive heart failure in patients who have received prior doxorubicin-containing regimens or in combination with doxorubicin. Left ventricular function should be evaluated in patients prior to and during treatment with trastuzumab.*

> *See Table 12-2.*

❖ Symptom Management

+ Side effects are similar to adjuvant chemotherapy and include neutropenia, nausea and vomiting, weight gain, alopecia, fatigue, arthralgias, and myalgias.

TABLE 12-2

Targeted Therapy in Metastatic Breast Cancer

Trastuzumab (Herceptin)

Mechanism of action	Recombinant humanized monoclonal anti-HER-2 antibody
	Targets extracellular domain of HER-2 growth factor receptor
	Inhibits signal transduction and cell proliferation
Indications/Use	Overexpression/amplification of HER-2/neu (c-erbB-2) metastatic breast cancer
Range of dosage	4 mg/kg IV loading dose over 90 minutes; then 2 mg/kg IV over 30 minutes weekly
Special precautions	During first infusion, mild to moderate chills and fever that usually abates with subsequent treatment
	Cardiotoxicity is a rare complication and may occur in patients previously treated with anthracyclines
Toxicity	Nausea and vomiting, pain are infrequent side effects
	Other side effects include increased anemia, leukopenia, diarrhea, and infection

+ The reader is referred to Chapter 10 for discussion of side effects and their management.

❖ **Nursing Management in Recurrent and Metastatic Breast Cancer**[14]

+ Help patient and family plan and assist in the scheduling of treatments to maintain level of functioning with the least amount of disruption.

◆ Understand the dilemmas facing women with advanced disease.

  Restart course of treatment

  Manage side effects

  Face major changes in role responsibilities at home and at work

  Face the difficulties of a shortened life expectancy

  Manage an uncertain future

◆ Explain treatment side effects.

◆ Provide emotional support and strengthening coping abilities.

  Help spouses, significant others, children, and other family members understand issues in advanced breast cancer.

  Refer to supportive networks, groups, and social workers.

REFERENCES

1. Ellis, M., Hayes, D., & Lippman, M. Treatment of metastatic breast cancer. In: J. R. Harris, M. Lippman, M. Morrow, C. K. Osborne (Eds.), *Diseases of the breast* (2nd ed., pp. 749–797). Philadelphia: Lippincott Williams & Wilkins.

2. Nabholtz, J. M., Mackey, J. R., Smylie, M., et al. (2001). Phase II study of docetaxel, doxorubicin, and

cyclophosphamide as first-line chemotherapy for metastatic breast cancer. *Journal of Clinical Oncology, 19,* 314–321.

3. Pagani, O., Sessa, C., Nole, F., et al. (2000). Epidoxorubicin and docetaxel as first-line chemotherapy in patients with advanced breast cancer: A multicentric phase I-II study. *Annals of Oncology, 11*(8), 985–991.

4. Miller, K. D., Sisk, J., Ansari, R., et al. (2001). Gemcitabine, paclitaxel, and trastuzumab in metastatic breast cancer. *Oncology, 15*(2 Suppl 3), 38–40.

5. Ibrahim, N. K., Buzdar, A. U., Valero, V., et al. (2001). Phase I study of vinorelbine and paclitaxel by 3-hour simultaneous infusion with and without granulocyte colony-stimulating factor support in metastatic breast carcinoma. *Cancer, 91,* 664–671.

6. Seidman, A. (2001). The evolving role of gemcitabine in the management of breast cancer. *Oncology, 60,* 189–198.

7. Hortobagyi, G. N. (2001). Treatment of advanced breast cancer with gemcitabine and vinorelbine. *Oncology* (Huntington), *15*(2 Suppl 3), 15–17.

8. Gradishar, W. J. (2001). Clinical status of capecitabine in the treatment of breast cancer. *Oncology* (Huntington) *15*(1Suppl 2), 69–71.

9. Perry, M. C., Anderson, C., Dorr, V., & Wilkes, J. (1999). *Companion Handbook to the Chemotherapy Sourcebook.* Philadelphia: Lippincott Williams & Wilkins.

10. Skeel, R. (1999). *Handbook of Cancer Chemotherapy,* 5th edition. Philadelphia: Lippincott Williams & Wilkins.

11. Wilkes, G., Ingwersen, K., Barton-Burke, M. (2000). *2000 Oncology Nursing Drug Handbook.* Sudbury, MA: Jones & Bartlett.

12. Slamon, D. J., Leyland-Jones, B., Shak, S., et al. (2001). Use of chemotherapy plus a monoclonal antibody against HER2 for metastatic breast cancer that overexpresses HER2. *New England Journal of Medicine, 344*(11), 783–892.

13. Fornier, M., Esteva, F., & Seidman, A. (2000). Trastuzumab in combination with chemotherapy for the treatment of metastatic breast cancer. *Seminars in Oncology, 6*(Suppl 11), 38–45.

14. Barse, P. (2000). Issues in the treatment of metastatic breast cancer. *Seminars in Oncology Nursing, 16*, 197–205.

13

Endocrine Therapy in Recurrent and Metastatic Disease

❖ Background[1]

+ Beatson observed regression of breast cancer after oophorectomy in 1896 and published the first paper on estrogen-dependent breast cancer.

+ Ablative procedures to remove ovaries and endocrine organs resulted in oophorectomy, adrenalectomy, and hypophysectomy, but there was high morbidity associated with surgery.

+ In the 1960s, pharmacologic approaches replaced ablative procedures with estrogens such as diethylstilbestrol (DES), and conjugated estrogens were the first agents used.

Major side effects, such as nausea, vomiting, uterine bleeding, edema, thrombolytic event, and

> *congestive heart failure, limited the use of early pharmacologic agents.*

> *Other endocrine therapy replaced the use of estrogens in metastatic breast cancer.*

+ Selection of patients for endocrine therapy is individualized.

+ Patients most likely to respond to endocrine therapy include the following:

   > *Those with estrogen receptor (ER)-positive and/or progesterone receptor (PR)-positive tumor*

   > *Disease-free interval greater than 2 years*

   > *Disease limited to bone and soft tissue*

   > *Asymptomatic visceral disease*

   > *Postmenopausal or late premenopausal status*

   > *Prior response to endocrine therapy*

+ Palliation is the principal goal of endocrine therapy.

+ First-line endocrine therapy

   > *Tamoxifen is the first-line endocrine therapy for both postmenopausal and premenopausal women because of its safety and tolerability.*

   > *Toremifene is also indicated as first-line endocrine treatment for metastatic disease.*

+ Second-line endocrine therapy

    With disease progression on tamoxifen, premenopausal women have estrogen-deprivation therapy with either luteinizing hormone–releasing hormone agonists (LH-RH) or oophorectomy.

    With disease progression on tamoxifen, postmenopausal women may be given selective aromatase inhibitors.

+ Third-line endocrine therapy

    With disease progression, other agents, such as megestrol acetate, estrogen/DES, androgen/ fluoxymestrone, and selective aromatase inhibitor (SAI) (if patient is SAI naïve), are used.

❖ **Tamoxifen**

+ Synthetic nonsteroidal triphenylethylene antiestrogen that binds to ER

+ Demonstrates mixed agonist/antagonist activity

+ Patients achieve good palliation with tamoxifen.

+ Mean time to disease progression for patients on tamoxifen is 6 months, with a duration of response of 12 to 18 months and up to several years.

+ Serious complications include thromboembolic events, endometrial cancer, pulmonary embolism, and cataracts.

> *Side effects include hot flashes, nausea, and vaginal discharge; potential depression*

+ Other antiestrogens with mixed agonists/ antagonists profiles

    Toremifine

    Idoxifene

    Droloxifene

    Raloxifene

❖ **Pure Antiestrogens[2]**

+ No agonist properties

+ Downregulates the estrogen receptor and is active in tamoxifen-resistant disease

+ Faslodex is given as an intramuscular agent

+ EM800

❖ **Aromatase Inhibitors[3]**

+ In postmenopausal women, estrogen synthesis in nongonadal sites increases. Peripheral tissue depends on the aromatization of androgenic precursors of adrenal origin (testosterone and androstenedione) to generate estradiol and estrone.

+ Aromatase is responsible for converting androgens to estrogens.

+ SAIs that suppress postmenopausal estrogen by

inhibiting the aromatase enzyme are more effective approaches, compared with non-SAIs such as aminoglutethimide.

> *Anastrozole (1 mg PO qd) and Letrozole (2.5 mg PO) are approved in the United States.*

> *SAI suppresses estradiol and estrone without a compensatory rise in androstenedione levels.*

> *Side effects include fatigue, headache, hot flashes, and gastrointestinal disturbance (e.g., nausea, vomiting, diarrhea).*

+ Steroidal aromatase inhibitors are an alternative to nonsteroidal inhibition of aromatase, with lack of cross-resistance with other aromatase inhibitors.

> *These agents bind aromatase and block the conversion of androgenic substrates.*

> *Exemestane, 25 mg PO, side effects include hot flashes, skin rash, lethargy, nausea, fatigue, anorexia, headache, and thromboembolic events.*

> *Formestane is another steroidal aromatase inhibitor but is not approved in the United States.*

❖ Luteinizing Hormone–Releasing Hormone Agonists[4]

+ LH-RH agonists are an alternative to oophorectomy for premenopausal women.

+ Goserelin and leuprolide are peptide analogues of

LRH that are up to 100 times more potent than the natural hormone.

+ LH-RH agonists stimulate follicle-stimulating hormone and luteinizing hormone secretion and affect the pituitary ovarian axis, with a fall in estrogen to menopausal levels.

+ LH-RH agonists have been combined with tamoxifen as first-line therapy in premenopausal women with metastatic disease, but the overall survival benefit is small.

❖ Progestins

+ Mechanism of action is unknown but may involve direct action on the cell mediated through progesterone and androgen receptor sites.

+ Indicated as third-line endocrine therapy in postmenopausal women, with an efficacy similar to that of tamoxifen.

+ Side effects include hypertension, weight gain, fluid retention, vaginal bleeding, and thromboembolic events.

❖ Management of Side Effects[5]

+ Nurses often regard endocrine therapy as somewhat "benign," compared with chemotherapy. However, patients experience side effects and are facing metastatic disease.

- Patient preparation for side effects and management
- Hot flashes are a major source of distress. The reader is referred to Chapter 17 for further discussion of the management of hot flashes.
- Changes in vaginal secretion: vaginal dryness, thinning, and dyspareunia
- Body image and mood disturbances and self-care management

REFERENCES

1. Ellis, M., Hayes, D., & Lippman, M. (2000). Treatment of metastatic breast cancer. In J. R. Harris, M. Lippman, M. Morrow, C. K. Osborne (Eds.), *Diseases of the breast* (2nd ed., pp. 749–797). Philadelphia: Lippincott Williams and Wilkins.

2. Howell, A., Osborne, C. K. Morris, C., & Wakeling, A. E. (2000). ICI 182, 780 (Faslodex): Development of a novel, "pure" antiestrogen. *Cancer, 89,* 817–825.

3. Buzdar, A. (2000). An overview of the use of non-steroidal aromatase inhibitors in the treatment of breast cancer. *European Journal of Cancer, 36* (Suppl 4), S82–S84.

4. Kimmick, G. G., & Muss, H. B. (1998). Endocrine therapy in metastatic breast cancer. *Cancer Treatment and Research, 94,* 231–254.

5. Cloutier, A. (2000). Advanced breast cancer: Recent developments in hormonal therapy. *Seminars in Oncology Nursing, 16,* 206–213.

PART IV

Quality-of-Life Issues in Breast Cancer

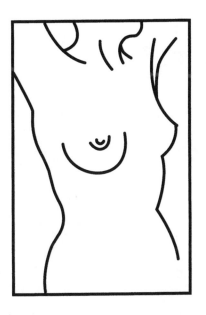

14

Late Physical Effects of Cancer Treatment

❖ **Long-Term Late Complications of Adjuvant Systemic Therapy**[1]

❖ **Cardiac Dysfunction**

✦ Cardiomyopathy may occur shortly after treatment ends or many months later.

✦ Incidence of congestive heart failure (CHF) in patients with doxorubicin-based chemotherapy varies based on total cumulative dose.

> *Standard four cycles of doxorubicin (A) and cyclophosphamide (C) with maximum total dose of doxorubicin 240 mg/m² did not demonstrate an increase in CHF.*

> *When total cumulative dose of doxorubicin is less than 300 mg/m², there is less incidence of cardiomyopathy.*

❖ **Amenorrhea and Ovarian Failure**

+ Incidence is about 70% in premenopausal and perimenopausal women, although it varies according to patient age, dose, and alkylating agent used.

+ Permanent ovarian dysfunction occurs in women over the age of 45.

+ Permanent ovarian dysfunction is less common in women under age 35.

+ Reader is referred to Chapters 17 and 18 for discussion about menopausal symptoms and reproductive effects, respectively.

❖ **Secondary Cancer**

+ Increased risk of myeloproliferative disease and acute leukemia is related to cumulative dose of the alkylating agent.

+ Leukemia risk is higher with the use of melphalan on prolonged treatment regimens.

❖ **Long-Term Late Physical Complications of Radiation Therapy[2]**

+ Long-term late physical complications of radiation therapy (XRT) may occur many years after treatment. While late complications are possible, their occurrence is rare.

+ Late complications

    Brachial plexopathy

    Soft-tissue necrosis

    Rib fractures

    Radiation pneumonitis

    Carcinogenesis (second breast cancer and soft-tissue sarcoma)

    Radiation-related cardiac disease

❖ **Brachial Plexopathy**

+ Extremely rare late physical effect

+ Occurs as a result of XRT to axillary and supraclavicular nodal regions

+ This injury is radiation dose-related and rarely occurs with doses less than 50 Gy delivered over 5 weeks (e.g., 56 Gy in 15 fractions to the axilla have higher risk of brachial plexopathy).

+ Signs and symptoms

    Mild discomfort in the shoulder and arm

    Paresthesias and weakness in the arm and hand that are progressive

    Evidence of soft-tissue fibrosis in supraclavicular and infraclavicular regions

    Difficult for clinicians to differentiate this brachial plexopathy from recurrence

+ Reversible brachial plexopathy

    Occurs at radiation doses less than 50 Gy and has a short latency period, with a median of about 4.5 months

+ There is no recognized therapy for brachial plexopathy.

❖ **Soft-Tissue Necrosis**

+ Soft-tissue necrosis is associated with postoperative XRT.

+ Patients older than 60 years are at higher risk.

+ This late effect rarely occurs today with modern radiation techniques and dose fractionation, but incidence increases with higher radiation dose or changes in fractionation schedules.

❖ **Rib Fractures**

+ Occur in the radiated field in 1% of patients, with a median time to occurrence of about 12 months

+ Rib fractures occur more often in patients treated with 4-meV (million electron volt) radiation treatment machines, compared with 6-meV or 8-meV treatment machines, and are most likely related to increased radiation dose to the lateral rib cage.

+ Other risk factors for rib fractures

    Prior trauma to this area

    Adjuvant chemotherapy

- ✦ Rib fracture does not necessarily represent bony metastases.

- ✦ Rib fractures are generally asymptomatic or associated with mild discomfort.

- ✦ Treatment with nonnarcotic analgesics and antiinflammatory agents.

❖ **Radiation Pneumonitis**

- ✦ Occurs in 1% of patients about 6 to 18 months after treatment

- ✦ Symptoms are generally transient.

    Dry cough

    Low-grade fever

    Shortness of breath

- ✦ Risk factors

    XRT to the supraclavicular region and axillary nodal region

    Three-field rather than two-field radiation

    Amount of lung irradiated

    Concurrent chemotherapy

❖ **Secondary Cancers**

- ✦ Contralateral breast cancer and sarcoma may occur after XRT for breast cancer.

    Latency period between exposure and detection is about 10 years.

> *Risk of carcinogenesis increases with doses up to 10 Gy and then levels off and declines.*
>
> *Dose to the opposite, unaffected breast is about 1 to 3 Gy and, thus, tumor induction in the ipsilateral breast may occur.*
>
> *Risk also increases when radiation is given at a younger age (less than 40 years).*

✦ Soft-tissue sarcoma

> *Rare complication that occurred in patients with mastectomy and postoperative XRT*

❖ **Cardiac Complications**

✦ Injury to heart is related to older radiation techniques, with higher radiation dose to the heart.

✦ Potential for XRT to increase risk of cardiomyopathy in patients treated with doxorubicin

REFERENCES

1. Osborne, C. K., & Ravdin, P. (2000). Adjuvant systemic therapy of primary breast cancer. In J. R. Harris, M. Lippman, M. Morrow, & C. K. Osborne (Eds.), *Diseases of the breast* (2nd ed., pp. 599–632). Philadelphia: Lippincott Williams and Wilkins.

2. Morrow, M., & Harris, J. R. (2000). Primary treatment of invasive breast cancer. In J. R. Harris, M. Lippman, M. Morrow, & C. K. Osborne (Eds.), *Diseases of the breast* (2nd ed., pp. 515–560). Philadelphia: Lippincott Williams and Wilkins.

15

Cancer-Related Fatigue and Sleep Disturbance

❖ **Cancer-Related Fatigue (CRF)**

  ✦ Most common side effect of cancer

  ✦ More distressing than nausea and vomiting

  ✦ Multidimensional experience relating to multiple and interacting causes

  ✦ Acute and/or chronic fatigue can occur over time.

  ✦ Specific mechanisms unknown

  ✦ Patterns of fatigue may be cyclic and cumulative

❖ **Patient Description of CRF**

  ✦ Physical sensation

    Dog-tired, bone-tired, weak, no strength, exhausted, no energy, drained, pooped

  ✦ Cognitive sensation

    Can't concentrate, confused, forgetful, distracted

+ Affective sensation

    Sadness, listless, decreased motivation

❖ Problems Associated with CRF

+ Influences sense of well-being

+ Change in daily performance

+ Change in activities of daily living

+ Change in relationships with family and friends

+ Change in work-related activities

+ Affects compliance with treatment

❖ Etiology of Fatigue in Breast Cancer

+ Surgical intervention

    Postoperative fatigue may be self-limiting.

    Other side effects from surgery, such as limited range of arm motion and pain, may increase the experience of fatigue.

    Acute and chronic lymphedema may contribute to fatigue.

+ Radiation therapy

    Pattern of fatigue in radiation therapy is progressive and increases during the course of treatment.

    Radiation side effects, such as skin reactions, may contribute to fatigue patterns, even when there is no change in red blood cell count.

+ Adjuvant chemotherapy[1,2]

  Treatment-related side effects, such as neutropenia, nausea, vomiting, weight gain, skin changes, nutritional pattern changes, and stomatitis, contribute to fatigue.

  Symptom cluster of sleep disturbances, anxiety, and depression may also contribute to the experience of fatigue.

❖ **Fatigue Models of Assessment[3]**

  + Piper Integrated Model of CRF

    Life event patterns

    Social patterns

    Environmental

    Psychological

    Change in regulation

    Oxygenation

    Activity/rest

    Sleep/wake

    Innate host factors

    Accumulation of metabolites

    Changes in energy

    Disease

    Treatment

    Symptom patterns

✦ Winningham Psychobiologic-Entropy Model[4]

   Correlates fatigue, symptoms, and functional status

   The cause of activity is less critical than the outcome of the decreased activity.

   Four propositions:

   1. Too much/little rest results in fatigue.

   2. Too little/much activity

   3. Balance needed between rest and activity

   4. Symptoms lead to less activity, more fatigue.

❖ Assessment of CRF[5,6]

+ Clinical assessment can be modeled on the approach to cancer pain assessment by asking, "On a scale of 0 to 10, where 0 is no fatigue and 10 is the most fatigue possible, how much fatigue do you have today?"

+ Assess for anemia

+ Assess fatigue patterns

+ Onset, duration, intensity, aggravating factors

+ Assess changes in usual activities

+ What changes have you made in your everyday activities?

+ Treatment history and current medication

+ Assess for and differentiate from depression and sadness

+ Assessment questions

  How much/little sleep do you get?

  What are your eating patterns?

  How are you feeling? Managing?

  Compliance with treatment?

  How well are you doing at work?

  What financial concerns do you have?

  Check for other contributing factors

  What was the pattern of fatigue, if any, before cancer and treatment?

+ Table 15-1 outlines differences between fatigue and depression.

Table 15-1
Differentiate Fatigue from Depression

Fatigue	Depression
Identifiable cause, such as anemia and infection	No identified cause
Cause may be treatable	No discernible pattern of fatigue
Pattern is related to cancer treatment	Intensity, pattern, and duration of sadness meet standard definition of depression

❖ Behavioral CRF Interventions[7]

+ Conserve energy and manage activities.

  Energy conservation techniques have been used in patients with physical illness.

  There are no standard guidelines for energy conservation in patients with cancer.

  Current suggestions are to prioritize activities that are either essential or nonessential.

  Determine level of attentional fatigue and plan attention-restoring activities.

  Plan and pace activities.

+ Promote rest and sleep.[8]

+ Nutritional support

  Early nutritional intervention, focusing on high-protein caloric intake

+ Alternative therapy

  Relaxation techniques, biofeedback, and massage therapy have been suggested and may be a promising intervention, but there are no controlled studies available to evaluate their effectiveness.

❖ Pharmacologic CRF Interventions

+ Management of cancer-related anemia

  Recombinant human erythropoietin (r-HuEPO) is a recognized and effective approach to treating anemia.

+ Psychostimulants

    Methylphenidate has been used, but there is no demonstrated efficacy of this drug in clinical trials.

❖ Exercise as an Intervention for Fatigue

+ National Comprehensive Cancer Network (NCCN) guidelines recommend exercise as the nonpharmacologic intervention having the strongest evidence of effectiveness.

+ Types of exercise include home-based walking programs and exercise cycles in the laboratory or hospital setting.

+ A review of studies indicate significantly lower levels of fatigue in individuals who exercise, compared with randomized control subjects.[9]

    Study outcomes also demonstrate increased performance, decreased anxiety and depression, and improved quality of life.

❖ The Exercise Prescription

+ General program

    Begin range of motion (ROM)/flexibility exercises and muscle strengthening, to maximize joint ROM and muscle endurance.

    Follow by submaximal aerobic exercise to enhance cardiopulmonary endurance.

+ Three basic components of an exercise program are frequency, intensity, and duration.

+ *Frequency* involves the number of exercises performed or number of walks per week.

> *Beginning exercisers are advised to exercise 4 to 6 days per week, not skipping more than 1 day in a row, and being certain to take 1 rest day every week.*

> *It is better to exercise for more frequent, short time periods than to exercise for longer periods, but less frequently.*

+ *Intensity* refers to how difficult the exercise is, difficulty being determined by the heart rate.

> *Women in an exercise program should be taught to take their pulse for 60 seconds while resting, to assess rate and rhythm.*

> *During exercise, the peak pulse just before the cool-down period is best measured by counting the pulse for 6 seconds and multiplying by 10.*

> *Because the pulse drops quickly when the individual stops exercising to measure it, the 6-second monitoring check best captures the peak pulse rate.*

> *As an intensity guide, rating of perceived exertion is a helpful adjunct to heart rate.*

+ *Duration:* The length of the exercise period is initially determined by the usual activity level of the individual.

    Begin gradually with a 5- or 10-minute brisk walk, always beginning (to warm up) and ending (to cool down) with several minutes of slow walking.

❖ **Precautions in an Exercise Program**

+ Wear comfortable, supportive shoes made specifically for walking or running.

+ Exercise in safe areas and preferably with an exercise partner.

+ Carry an emergency card.

+ Maintain hydration.

❖ **Contraindications to Exercise**

+ No exercise on the days of chemotherapy administration

+ No exercise before blood drawing to check laboratory values

+ No exercise if any of the following laboratory values are present:

    White blood cell count less than 3,000 μL

    Absolute neutrophil count less than 2,500 μL

    Hemoglobin/hematocrit less than 10 g/dL

    Platelet count less than 25,000 μL

+ Do not exercise if there is metastatic bone involvement of greater than 25% of the cortex.

+ High-impact aerobics are contraindicated during chemotherapy and in recurrent disease.

+ Presence of fever

+ Resume exercise carefully following illness, surgery, or new treatment protocols.

❖ **Adherence to an Exercise Program**

+ Exercise is a learned behavior; the first goal should be to establish the habit of exercise.

+ Incorporate effective behavioral strategies to encourage adherence.

+ Women with breast cancer are often highly motivated to do whatever they can to improve their health.

+ Regular reinforcement by supportive friends and family members, and members of the health care team, can help sustain the patient's commitment.

+ Encourage the patient to keep an exercise diary, which offers a patient the reward of seeing her progress over time and may help reinforce the exercise habit.

+ Encourage the patient to exercise with a committed friend or family member.

+ Some individuals prefer group exercise and find that this enhances their adherence.

+ Exercise should be enjoyable; examples include walking, jogging, swimming, and biking.

+ Schedule the exercise period as a part of one's daily activities and at a convenient time and location.

❖ **Self-Paced Walking Exercise Program**

+ Allows for periods of decreased performance due to effects of the disease or treatment.

+ Should be modest enough for the individual to feel successful versus an intensive program, which leaves an individual feeling sore and exhausted

❖ **Sleep Disturbance[10]**

+ Sleep disturbance and mood disturbance often accompany fatigue.

+ Sleep problems are a common side effect; however, there are few empirical data on management available.

+ Sleep problems are categorized as insomnia (inability to sleep) or hypersomnia (inability to maintain wakefulness).

+ Chronic sleep problems may lead to difficulty concentrating or paying attention, irritability, and depression.

+ Assessment of sleep disturbance is complex.

Determine differences in current level of sleep patterns, compared with that before treatment.

What is the quality and quantity of sleep since the cancer diagnosis?

Keep a sleep log to record time of sleep onset, duration of sleep, sleep habits, frequency and reason for awakening, naps, and use of sleep aids.

What are the patterns of insomnia (sleep onset, wakenings)?

What are the present pre-sleep routines? Daily activities?

What are the environmental considerations in sleep (noise, light, room temperature)?

Are there any physiologic problems present that can interfere with sleep? (pain, dyspnea, hot flashes)

What food and medications may be interfering with sleep? (caffeine, alcohol)

What are the emotional factors to consider?

+ Management of sleep disturbance

Two categories: nonpharmacologic and pharmacologic

+ Non-pharmacologic management

Establish sleep ritual: time for sleep and awakening every day.

Avoid stimulants (e.g., caffeine, chocolate, nicotine), alcohol, heavy meals, and exercise just prior to sleep.

Take a warm bath or shower before sleep.

Exercise regularly to improve sleep.

Control of other symptoms and side effects of treatment.

Behavioral relaxation, including progressive muscle relaxation training, passive muscle relaxation training, meditation, hypnosis, and guided imagery

Cognitive control techniques, including counting, cognitive refocusing, guided imagery, and ocular relaxation

+ Pharmacologic intervention

Benzodiazepines

Nonbarbiturate, nonbenzodiazepine (chloral hydrate)

Antidepressants

Antihistamines

❖ **Website Resources**

+ CancerFatigue.org at http://www.cancerfatigue.org

+ FatigueNet at http://www.fatiguenet.com

REFERENCES

1. Broeckel, J., Jacobsen, P., Horton, J., et al. (1998). Characteristics and correlates of fatigue after adjuvant

chemotherapy for breast cancer. *Journal of Clinical Oncology, 16*, 1689–1696.

2. Berger, A., & Higginbotham, P. (2000). Correlates of fatigue during and following adjuvant breast cancer chemotherapy: A pilot study. *Oncology Nursing Forum, 27*, 1443–1448.

3. Piper, B., Dibble, S., Dodd, M., et al. (1998). The Revised Piper Fatigue Scale: Psychometric evaluation in women with breast cancer. *Oncology Nursing Forum, 25,* 677–684.

4. Winningham, M. (1999). Fatigue. In C. H. Yarbro, M. H. Frogge, & M. Goodman (Eds.), *Cancer symptom management* (2nd ed., pp. 58–76). Sudbury, MA: Jones and Bartlett.

5. Nail, L. (1997). Fatigue. In R. Gates & R. Fink (Eds.), *Oncology nursing secrets* (pp. 234–239). Philadelphia: Hanley and Belfus.

6. Berger, A., & Farr, L. (1999). The influence of daytime inactivity and nighttime restlessness on cancer-related fatigue. *Oncology Nursing Forum, 26,* 1663–1671.

7. Buchsel, P., Barton-Burke, M., & Winningham, M. (2000). Treatment: An overview. In M. Winningham & M. Barton-Burke (Eds.), *Fatigue in cancer: A multidimensional approach* (pp. 153–179). Sudbury, MA: Jones and Bartlett.

8. Owen, D., Parker, K., & McGuire, D. (1999). Comparison of subjective sleep quality in patients with cancer and healthy subjects. *Oncology Nursing Forum, 26,* 1649–1651.

9. Mock, V. (2001). Exercise to mitigate cancer-related fatigue: A critique of the research with directions for future studies (abstract). Proceedings of the Sixth National Conference on Cancer Nursing Research, Oncology Nursing Society, p. 78.

10. Yellen, S., & Dyonzak, J. (1999). Sleep. In C. H. Yarbro, M. H. Frogge, & M. Goodman (Eds.), *Cancer symptom management* (2nd ed., pp. 161–197). Sudbury, MA: Jones and Bartlett.

16

Lymphedema

+ Lymphedema is an abnormal collection of excessive tissue proteins, edema, chronic inflammation, and fibrosis that occurs from an imbalance between fluid deposited in tissue and the ability of the lymphatic system to handle the fluid. It is the result of a functional overload of the lymphatic system in which lymph volume exceeds transport capabilities.

❖ **Problems with Lymphedema**

+ A troublesome complication

+ No known cure for lymphedema

+ Swelling can be painful.

+ Restriction of arm movement can limit activities of daily living.

+ Lymphedema is a recognized complication of breast cancer treatment that affects approximately 20% of patients.[1] Despite the decline in the use of mastectomy, the incidence continues. There may be underreporting of this complication for several reasons.[2]

❖ Factors Relating to Underreporting of Lymphedema

+ Onset may be gradual over several years.

+ Lymphedema has not been considered a "life-threatening" complication.

+ There is a lack of standard reporting and measuring criteria for lymphedema.

❖ Types of Lymphedema

+ *Acute* lymphedema lasts between 3 and 6 months and has a pitting quality.

  Excess fluid is accommodated by a large subcutaneous tissue space that can expand.

  Noticeable fluctuations in arm size are typical, with the largest increase noted at night.

+ *Chronic* lymphedema lasts longer than 6 months.

  Affected skin becomes hard, thick, and brawny in appearance.

  Change occurs over time as fluid becomes embedded in subcutaneous connective tissues, restricting joint movement.

❖ Categories of Lymphedema

+ Grade I: Pitting occurs with applying pressure, and edema reverses with limb elevation.

+ Grade II: Edema becomes larger and harder and does not pit under pressure.

+ Grade III: Swelling worsens and skin changes occur; skin becomes thick and develops folds, with elephantiasis.

❖ **Pathophysiology of Lymphedema in Breast Cancer**

+ Lymphedema associated with breast cancer is considered secondary lymphedema caused by mechanical obstruction of lymphatic channels after surgery and radiation therapy.

> *Reader is referred to Chapter 6 on surgical techniques for additional information about axillary lymph node dissection (ALND).*

> *ALND of level I, II, and III nodes is the greatest contributor to development of lymphedema.*

> *Level I nodes are located at the tail of the breast.*

> *Level II nodes are closest to the breast and drain the breast area.*

> *Level III nodes are located between the pectoralis muscle along subscapular vessels and the chest wall.*

> *Sentinel lymph node biopsy (SLNB) is being evaluated as a diagnostic alternative to ALND and is associated with a decreased incidence of lymphedema.*

+ Radiation therapy to the axilla increases the risk of lymphedema.

    Incidence of lymphedema is highest when both ALND and axillary radiation are performed.

    While lymphatic vessels are resistant to radiation, lymph nodes are sensitive and go through a process of reduced lymphocytes, fatty tissue replacement, and localized fibrosis.

❖ Risk Factors for Lymphedema[3]

+ Extent of ALND and axillary radiation therapy

+ Older age at diagnosis

+ Postoperative infection

+ Obesity

❖ Symptoms Co-occurring with Lymphedema

+ Pain

    Pain is related to nerve damage during surgery; postmastectomy pain syndrome

    Stretching of tissue, which accommodates the build-up of lymph fluid

    When the fluid increases, the arm becomes visibly swollen and feels heavy, with an increase in arm size.

+ Range of motion (ROM) restrictions of ipsilateral arm

    Result of tissue manipulation and positioning during surgery

    Lymphedema also causes ROM restrictions in the shoulder, elbow, and wrist.

+ Sensation changes

    Sensation changes may be related to surgical incision or to nerve irritation or injury during ALND.

    Sensations include phantom breast sensations, numbness, hyperesthesias, and "pins and needles" sensations.

    Dysesthesia is described as a cutting or burning pain.

❖ **Psychosocial Issues Related to Lymphedema**

+ Depression and anxiety relating to functional impairment

+ Body image concerns relating to appearance of arm

+ Increased feeling of social isolation

❖ **Diagnosis of Lymphedema**

+ Physical examination with findings of a greater than 2-cm difference between affected and contralateral limb circumferences.

Women often present with a feeling of tightness in clothing or jewelry.

Location, quality, intensity, duration, precipitating, and alleviating factors related to the swelling

Arm size measurement using circumferential arm measures at various points (i.e., 1–20 points measured every 5–10 cm) along the involved extremity compared with the uninvolved extremity is highly subjective.

+ Lymphatic imaging has also been used.

+ Absence of standard measurement with acceptable reliability and validity, lack of uniform definition, and evaluation of treatments limit the diagnosis of lymphedema.

❖ **Prevention of Lymphedema**

+ Prevention is the major goal, because there is no cure for lymphedema.

+ Focus of prevention is minimizing injury or damage to the involved extremity.

+ Precautions recommended by National Lymphedema Network[4]

Do not ignore any swelling.

Do not allow injection or blood draw in the affected arm.

Check blood pressure on the unaffected arm.

Maintain skin and nail care.

Avoid vigorous exercises using the affected arm.

Do not lift heavy objects with the affected arm.

Avoid excessive heat, saunas, sunburns, tans, and hot baths.

Do not wear constricting garments, jewelry, and sleeves.

Prevent arm swelling and infection.

Use sunscreen on the affected arm.

Wear gloves while doing housework.

Wear a compression sleeve during air travel.

Use an electric razor to remove axillary hair.

Maintain ideal body weight; avoid smoking and alcohol.

❖ Management of Lymphedema Using Complex Physical Therapy (CPT)

+ Four components and two phases of CPT

   Skin care

   Massage

   Compression bandaging

   Exercise

   Two phases of CPT, with the first phase lasting 4 to 6 weeks to establish lymphedema reduction and the second phase involving maintenance of initial reduction

+ Skin care

    Liberal use of lotions to keep arm moist and supple

    Use of oil-based soaps

    Avoidance of injury or even minor damage (e.g., bruises, sunburn, insect bites, abrasion, etc.) to the affected arm

+ Massage

    Manual lymphatic drainage or manual lymphatic therapy

    Goal is to empty truncal regions of the body first, with the proximal arm massaged before the distal arm.

    Massage is performed slowly, with minimal pressure and friction.

+ Compression bandaging

    Compression bandages applied immediately after massage

    Low-stretch, low-elastic bandages applied from distal to proximal areas

+ Exercise

    Exercises are sequenced to facilitate movement of fluid into the lymphatics.

> *Jarring or pounding exercises (e.g., tennis, softball)
> are not recommended.*

❖ **Other Treatment for Lymphedema**

  ✦ Diuretics

  ✦ Benzopyrones

❖ **Nursing Management**[5,6]

  ✦ Review lymphedema pathophysiology and
    prevention.

  ✦ Ask patients about lymphedema—patients may
    not volunteer information unless asked directly.

  ✦ Monitor patients closely when lymphedema
    occurs.

  ✦ Suggest that patients wear a medical alert bracelet.

  ✦ Do not dismiss even a seemingly minor injury.

REFERENCES

1. Petrek, J., Pressman, P., & Smith, R. (2000). Lymphedema:
   Current issues in research and management. *CA: Cancer
   Journal for Clinicians, 50,* 292–307.

2. Hull, M. (2000). Lymphedema in women treated for
   breast cancer. *Seminars in Oncology Nursing, 16* (3),
   226–237.

3. Erickson, V., Pearson, M., Ganz, P., et al. (2001). Arm
   edema in breast cancer patients. *Journal of the National
   Cancer Institute, 93,* 96–111.

4. Thiadens, S. (1999). 18 steps to prevention for arm lymphedema. National Lymphedema Network website available at: http://www.lymphnet.org/prevention.html

5. Kalinowski, B. Lymphedema. In C. H. Yarbro, M. H. Frogge, & M. Goodman (Eds.), *Cancer symptom management* (2nd ed., pp. 457–486). Sudbury, MA: Jones and Bartlett.

6. Coward, D. (1999). Lymphedema prevention and management knowledge in women treated for breast cancer. *Oncology Nursing Forum, 26,* 1047–1053.

17

Menopausal Symptoms

+ Menopausal symptoms[1] occurring as a result of breast cancer treatment have a significant effect on the quality of life of women.

+ Greater attention is being paid to menopausal symptoms and their relief.

❖ **Menopause**

+ Definition: Cessation of menses for 12 months

+ Average age of occurrence of natural menopause: 51 to 52 years (range: 40–60 years)

❖ **Changes Occurring during Menopause**

+ Morphologic change in the ovary and change in hormonal levels

+ Ovaries become smaller, fibrotic, and devoid of any functional follicle.

+ Estradiol, the dominant source of estrogen for the premenopausal woman, dramatically declines.

- ✦ Estrone becomes the principal source of estrogen for the postmenopausal woman.

- ✦ Levels of gonadotrophins (FSH, LH) rise significantly after menopause due to estrogen loss.

❖ **Menopause and Cancer**

- ✦ Artifically induced as a result of treatment

    Radiation therapy to the ovaries

    Surgical removal of the ovaries (i.e., oophorectomy)

    Chemotherapy produces gonadal toxicity (i.e., cyclophosphamide).

❖ **Target Tissues Affected**

- ✦ Vasomotor

- ✦ Skeletal system

- ✦ Cardiovascular system

- ✦ Urogenital tract

❖ **Vasomotor Symptoms: Hot Flashes**

- ✦ Most frequently occurring symptom of menopause, with up to 85% experiencing hot flashes

- ✦ Etiology of hot flashes is unknown but consists of both a subjective and physiologic component with estrogen withdrawal and disruption of thermoregulation and neuroendocrine pathways.

✦ Increased problem of hot flashes in women with breast cancer[2]

> *Women may have been on hormone replacement therapy (HRT) previously but must discontinue it after a breast cancer diagnosis and thus precipitate or exacerbate hot flashes.[3]*

> *Hot flashes and other menopausal symptoms are more frequent, severe, bothersome, and disruptive in women with breast cancer, compared with naturally premenopausal, perimenopausal, and postmenopausal women.[4]*

> *Hot flashes also can occur with tamoxifen therapy.*

> *Disruption of circadian rhythms of hormone and body temperature may also affect the severity of hot flashes.*

✦ Symptoms are unique to the individual.

> *Vary from transient episodes of feelings of warmth to episodes of intense overheating*

> *May be accompanied by sweats, palpitations, anxiety, and chills*

> *Patients may report experiencing a premonition or aura right before the hot flash.*

> *Heart rate and skin blood flow increase, and distribution of the heat sensation is to the upper body.*

> *Hot flashes occur at various times during a 24-hour period, with no particular established pattern.*

+ Key factor is the withdrawal of estrogen, not low estrogen level.

+ Other precipitating factors include ambient temperature, hot drinks and food, alcohol, caffeine, and emotional distress.

❖ **Pharmacologic Management of Hot Flashes[5]**

+ Venlafaxine is an antidepressant that affects serotonin and norepinephrine reuptake and has been effective in reducing hot flashes in a placebo-controlled clinical trial.[6]

> *Side effects increase with increasing the dose of venlafaxine from 37.5 mg to 75 mg to 150 mg/ day.*

> *Improvement in other symptoms, such as decreased tiredness and decreased sweating may occur.*

+ Clonidine is the most common alpha-adrenergic agonist used for the relief of hot flashes.

> *Low-dose clonidine (0.1 mg/day), administered either in pill form or by a transdermal patch, reduces the frequency and severity of vasomotor symptoms.*

> *Dose escalation is associated with improved response.*

> *Side effects of dizziness, nausea, dry mouth, and headache make higher doses unacceptable for some women.*

+ Bellergal (ergotamine tartrate), belladonna alkaloids, and phenobarbital have been used.

> *Potential addictive risk and the availability of safer alternatives limit the usefulness of these agents.*

+ Low-dose progestational agents have demonstrated some efficacy.

> *Medroxyprogesterone acetate (Provera)*

> *Megestrol acetate 20 mg (Megace)*

> *Progestins are associated with menstrual bleeding.*

> *Other side effects: breast tenderness, mood changes, and abdominal bloating, which may affect acceptability and adherence*

+ Vitamin E[7]

> *Limited effectiveness in decreasing hot flashes*

> *Recommended doses vary but are in the range of 200 to 800 mg/day.*

> *Also used as a lubricant or suppository to relieve vaginal dryness symptoms*

> *Women with heart disease, diabetes, or hypertension must consult their physicians before taking Vitamin E.*

> *Benefit: Vitamin E is an inexpensive medication.*

❖ **Nonpharmacologic Management of Hot Flashes**

✦ Behavioral strategies

Relaxation training, such as progressive muscle relaxation, may decrease sympathetic nervous system arousal.

Dietary changes, with avoidance of caffeine and alcohol and an increase in soy-based products

Regular physical exercise

Acupuncture is being evaluated in clinical studies

❖ **Skeletal Effects: Osteoporosis[8]**

✦ Reduction in bone mass, leading to osteoporosis

✦ Low bone mass with microarchitectural deterioration

✦ Increased risk of osteoporotic fractures of the distal forearm, spine, and hip

✦ Women with breast cancer are at higher risk of osteoporosis.

Women who receive chemotherapy experience premature menopause at an earlier age and with lower bone mineral density (BMD), compared with women not receiving chemotherapy[9]

Breast cancer survivors are not candidates for HRT and may lose up to 30% of bone mass within the first year of menopause without estrogen.

+ Other risk factors for osteoporosis

    Advancing age

    Family history

    Ethnicity, with White and Asian women having higher risk and African American and Hispanic women having lower risk

    Small body size and low body weight (less than 127 pounds)

+ Diagnosis of osteoporosis

    Bone mineral density studies, DEXA scan, repeated every 2 years

+ Pharmacologic management

    Estrogen replacement therapy, alendronate, and raloxifene are indicated to prevent and/or treat osteoporosis.

    Calcitonin is indicated for treatment of osteoporosis only.

    Estrogen/hormone replacement therapy is a treatment for osteoporosis but is generally contraindicated in women with breast cancer.

    Bisphosphonates reduce bone loss by inhibiting the action of osteoclasts, and reduce vertebral fractures.[10]

    Selective estrogen receptor modulators (SERMs) may augment bone mineral density.

Calcitonin is a naturally occurring hormone that is involved in calcium regulation and reduces bone loss in the spine.

+ Nonpharmacologic interventions

  Exercise 30 minutes a day, three times a week.

  Adhere to a weight-bearing, strength, and weight training program that is frequent and progressive in intensity.

  Improve environment to reduce the risk of falls (wear sturdy, low-heeled shoes; secure rugs in home).

+ Nutritional changes

  High-calcium diet, including dairy products (i.e., milk, yogurt, ice cream, cheese), fruits, vegetables (e.g., broccoli, legumes, kale), and tofu (i.e., soy, soy milk).

  Calcium supplements of 1,500 mg/day in divided doses of 500 mg, with Vitamin D 200 to 400 IU to help absorb calcium

  Do not take calcium supplements with caffeine, which can affect the absorption of calcium.

  Stop smoking and decrease alcohol intake.

+ Resources

  National Osteoporosis Foundation (NOF) is a nonprofit, voluntary health organization dedicated to reducing the prevalence of

*osteoporosis. Access is available at
http://www.nof.org*

❖ **Cardiovascular Effects**

✦ Cardiovascular disease is the leading cause of death in women in the United States.

✦ Risk of cardiovascular disease increases with estrogen deficiency.

✦ Estrogen has a protective cardiovascular effect. When estrogen is decreased, it causes changes in plasma total cholesterol and lipid profile.

✦ Decreased estrogen results in a higher level of low-density lipoprotein (LDL) cholesterol and a lower concentration of high-density lipoprotein (HDL) cholesterol.

✦ Other risk factors for cardiovascular disease

Obesity, hypertension, diabetes, sedentary lifestyle, cigarette smoking

✦ Management to reduce risk of cardiovascular disease

Stop smoking.

Exercise 30 minutes a day, three times a week.

Moderate diet to lower fat intake and control blood lipid levels.

Vitamin E, 400 to 800 units, has a protective effect against coronary artery disease (CAD).

> *Dietary supplements of folate plus Vitamin B6 and B12 reduce homocysteine levels and may decrease the risk for CAD.*
>
> *Aspirin, 75 to 325 mg per day, offers protection against CAD.*
>
> *Lipid- and cholesterol-modifying medications are prescribed for patients with an unfavorable profile.*

❖ **Urogenital Tract[11]**

◆ Atrophic changes in the vagina result in vaginal dryness, dyspareunia, and atrophic vaginitis.

◆ Urogenital atrophy and urinary symptoms include dysuria, frequency, urgency, nocturia, urinary stress incontinence, and urinary tract infections.

◆ Decrease in vaginal lubrication, atrophic vaginitis, and frequent infection can result in dyspareunia.

◆ Management

> *Water-soluble lubricants have been the historical intervention when estrogen (systemic or cream) is contraindicated.*
>
> *Vaginal lubricants: KY-jelly, Replens, and Astroglide*
>
> *Replens has been reported to increase vaginal moisture and elasticity and return vaginal pH to its premenopausal state.*

+ Management of urinary symptoms

    Kegel strengthening exercises

    Bladder training program: Void at regular time intervals.

    Promote adequate fluid intake.

❖ **Recommendations for Practice**

+ Informing the patient of the potential for drug-induced ovarian failure and menopausal symptoms

+ Routine follow-up assessment

+ Ovarian failure and associated symptoms may occur over several months.

+ Effects may not be evident until after adjuvant therapy is completed.

+ Discuss interventions and side effects.

+ Promote health-improving routines such as exercise and nutritional changes.

+ Discuss the risks and benefits of HRT.

REFERENCES

1. Swain, S., Sante, R., Burger, H., & Pritchard, K. (1999). Treatment of estrogen deficiency symptoms in women surviving breast cancer. Part 4: Urogenital atrophy,

vasomotor instability, sleep disorders, and related symptoms. *Oncology, 13,* 551–575.

2. Carpenter, J. (2000). Hot flashes and their management in breast cancer. *Seminars in Oncology Nursing, 16,* 214–225.

3. Snyder, G., Sielsch, E., & Reville, B. (1998). The controversy of hormone-replacement therapy in breast cancer survivors. *Oncology Nursing Forum, 25,* 699–706.

4. Carpenter, J. (2001). Hot flashes and other menopausal symptoms in breast cancer survivors and age-matched healthy comparison women (abstract). Proceedings of the Sixth National Conference on Cancer Nursing Research, Oncology Nursing Society, February 8–10, 2001, p. 102.

5. Cobleigh, M. (2000). Managing menopausal problems. In *Diseases of the breast* (2nd ed., pp. 1041–1050). J. R. Harris, M. Lippman, M. Morrow, & C. K. Osborne (Eds.), Philadelphia: Lippincott Williams & Wilkins.

6. Loprinzi, C. L., Kugler, J. W., Sloan, J. A., et al. (2000). Venlafaxine in management of hot flashes in survivors of breast cancer: A randomised controlled trial. *Lancet, 356* (9247), 2059–2063.

7. Barton, D., Loprinzi, C., Quella, S., et al. (1998). Prospective evaluation of vitamin E for hot flashes in breast cancer survivors. *Journal of Clinical Oncology, 16,* 495–500.

8. Mahon, S. M. (1998). Osteoporosis: A concern for cancer survivors. *Oncology Nursing Forum, 25,* 843–851.

9. Headley, J., Theriault, R., LeBlanc, A., et al. (1998). Pilot study of bone mineral density in breast cancer patients treated with adjuvant chemotherapy. *Cancer Investigation, 16,* 6–11.

10. Delmas, P., Balena, R., Confavreux, E., et al. (1997). Bisphosphonate risedronate prevents bone loss in women with artificial menopause due to chemotherapy of breast cancer: A double-blind, placebo-controlled study. *Journal of Clinical Oncology, 15,* 955–962.

11. Goodman, M. Menopausal symptoms. In C. H. Yarbro, M. H. Frogge, & M. Goodman (Eds.), *Cancer symptom management* (2nd ed., pp. 95–111). Sudbury, MA: Jones and Bartlett.

18

Reproductive Effects

❖ Overview

- ✦ Although the incidence of breast cancer in premenopausal women is less than 20%, the impact of treatment on fertility is a major distress and a significant quality-of-life concern.

- ✦ Advancing age and alkylating agents are known risk factors influencing fertility.

- ✦ Hormonal therapy and taxanes in adjuvant chemotherapy have increased length of treatment.

- ✦ Assisted reproductive technologies (ARTs) may also influence fertility and pregnancy outcomes in younger women.

❖ Impact of Cancer Treatment on Fertility

- ✦ Mastectomy

    No known effect on fertility

    Influence future ability of woman to breast-feed

+ Radiation therapy

    Contraindicated during pregnancy

    After treatment, may influence ability to breast-feed from irradiated breast

+ Chemotherapy

    Small fraction of ovarian follicles cycle during any one time, with the cycling cells most susceptible to damage from chemotherapy.[1]

    Cyclophosphamide-containing adjuvant therapy results in endocrine hormone profiles that are consistent with primary ovarian failure:

    1. Fall in estradiol and progesterone levels

    2. Elevation in follicle-stimulating hormone (FSH) and luteinizing hormone (LH) levels

    3. Increase in vaginal epithelial atrophy and endometrial hypoplasia

    Degree of amenorrhea is variable and is related to prolonged dosing, higher dose regimens, and total dose of cyclophosphamide.

    Doxorubicin does not appreciably increase the risk of amenorrhea when added to cyclophosphamide.

    Onset of amenorrhea is age related, with decreased likelihood of regaining menses after age 45 after adjuvant chemotherapy.

Anthracycline-based chemotherapy has less ovarian toxicity than cyclophosphamide, methotrexate, fluorouracil (CMF)-based chemotherapy.

✦ Tamoxifen

Use results in an increase in estradiol and total estrogen levels without a significant rise in FSH or LH.

When tamoxifen is added to adjuvant chemotherapy, the risk of amenorrhea rises in women over the age of 35.

Even when women do not experience amenorrhea with tamoxifen, they are on hormonal therapy for at least 5 years and cannot attempt pregnancy during tamoxifen treatment.

Women can get pregnant while on tamoxifen therapy and thus should use appropriate contraception.

Women should wait until 2 months after tamoxifen therapy before attempting pregnancy, due to the long half-life of tamoxifen.

✦ Taxane therapy

The effect of addition or substitution of taxanes in adjuvant chemotherapy on ovarian function is not yet known.

✦ Bone marrow transplantation is associated with a high rate of ovarian failure, and women who receive high-dose chemotherapy should expect permanent amenorrhea.

❖ **Chemotherapy Drugs in Breast Cancer Increasing Risk of Amenorrhea**

- ✦ Definite: cyclophosphamide

- ✦ Probable: doxorubicin

- ✦ Unlikely: methotrexate, 5-fluorouracil

❖ **Age as an Influencing Factor in Amenorrhea**

- ✦ Fertility rates decline significantly after age 41 in the normal population without breast cancer.

- ✦ Increasing age in combination with cyclophosphamide has an effect on development of amenorrhea.[2]

    Average cumulative dose of 5.2 g cyclophosphamide has resulted in amenorrhea among women in their 40s, compared with 9.3 g cyclophosphamide among women in their 30s.

    CMF (cyclophosphamide, methotrexate, fluorouracil): Amenorrhea in women age 40 years was 40%, compared with 76% in women over the age of 40[3]

    AC (doxorubicin and cyclophosphamide): No incidence of amenorrhea at 1 year after AC in women younger than age 45 years, compared with women over age 45 years

- ✦ Prolonged dosing can cause amenorrhea, even in younger women.

❖ Effects of Subsequent Pregnancy on Survival

- ◆ There have been no epidemiologic studies to date that have suggested an adverse effect of pregnancy on survival.

- ◆ Retrospective institutional reports conducted between 1940 and 1979, case-control studies conducted between 1965 and 1997, and population-based studies (1994–1999) have not shown an adverse effect on survival.

- ◆ Potential form of bias called "healthy mother effect" may explain why women who become pregnant may be more likely free of disease at the time of pregnancy, compared with women who do not have subsequent pregnancy.[4]

- ◆ Some studies suggest equal or improved survival in multiple pregnancies.

❖ Risk of Spontaneous Abortion after Breast Cancer

- ◆ Risk of spontaneous abortion was examined in one study.

- ◆ Rate of miscarriage was 24% among 53 women with breast cancer who became pregnant after diagnosis, compared with 18% in 265 case-matched control subjects who never had breast cancer.[5]

❖ Prevention of Treatment-Related Ovarian Failure

- ◆ Ovarian suppression using a gonadotropin-releasing hormone (GnRH) agonist has been used to reduce ovarian toxicity in other young cancer survivors.[6]

+ 94% of patients with lymphoma who received a GnRH agonist resumed normal menses, compared with 39% in the nonrandomized control group.

+ GnRH agonist use results in an initial stimulatory effect on the ovary, and in animal models, an LH-RH agonist can reduce cyclophosphamide-mediated depletion of ovarian follicles and preserve proliferative activity.

> *GnRH agonist must be started at least 7 to 10 days prior to the first chemotherapy session to ensure that ovarian suppression is achieved.*

+ Second option is the use of cyclic oral contraceptives in cancer patients with Hodgkin's disease, lymphoma, and germ-cell tumors, but the results are equivocal.

+ Third preventive option is to limit young women's overall exposure to alkylating agents, such as cyclophosphamide, to four cycles of AC.

❖ **Questions/Concerns about Pregnancy after Breast Cancer**

+ What is a reasonable amount of time to wait before attempting a pregnancy?

> *Each woman must feel psychologically and physically in shape after cancer treatment before starting a pregnancy.*

Suggestions from the literature are variable, with most suggesting a wait of at least 1 year.

Others recommend at least a 2-year wait, until the greatest risk of recurrence has passed. However, risk of recurrence can be up to 25 years after treatment.

Other quality-of-life considerations must be taken into account. For example, younger women who receive adjuvant chemotherapy and continue to menstruate are at higher risk for early menopause. If young women desire pregnancy, they need to consider pregnancy sooner rather than later, with reduced chances of conception.

✦ Will more than one pregnancy affect recurrence?

Limited data do not indicate that more than one pregnancy adversely influences recurrence.

✦ What is the safety in breast-feeding?

If a woman has received breast-conserving surgery and radiation therapy, there will be either diminished or absent milk production in the irradiated breast.

Radiation causes ductal shrinkage, condensation of cytoplasm lining the duct, atrophy of lobules, and perilobar and periductal fibrosis

✦ What is the health of children of women with breast cancer?

> *Evidence does not suggest an adverse effect on the health of infants born to mothers with a history of breast cancer.*

+ What circumstances may occur to suggest termination of pregnancy?

> *There are no easy answers, and there must be a highly individualized discussion.*

> *In situations in which a patient develops recurrence/ metastatic disease during the first trimester of pregnancy and must start adjuvant chemotherapy and/or radiation therapy, discussion of pregnancy termination is necessary.*

❖ Management of Treatment-Related Ovarian Failure

+ Techniques for oocyte cryopreservation have had limited success.

+ There are very limited data on the long-term effects of women who use ART.

+ Types of drugs used to stimulate ovarian production

> *Clomiphene citrate*

> *Human menopausal gonadotropin (hMG)*

> *Follicle-stimulating hormone (FSH)*

> *Gonadotropin-releasing hormone (GnRH) agonists*

+ Adverse effects with ART

> *Ovarian hyperstimulation syndrome (OHHS),*
>> *characterized by fluid accumulation in peritoneal,*
>> *pleural, and pericardial cavities*
>
> *Trabecular bone loss is dose and duration dependent,*
>> *with slow bone recovery.*
>
> *Adverse reproductive outcomes, including multiple*
>> *gestations*
>
> *Potential association in the use of fertility drugs and*
>> *risk of ovarian cancer, although this is*
>> *nonconclusive, based on several studies[7,8]*

- Clomiphene-induced ovulation followed by oocyte retrieval and in vitro fertilization (IVF) has been performed successfully in women who developed infertility after breast cancer.[9]

❖ Adoption as an Alternative to Pregnancy

- Women must come to terms with amenorrhea and infertility after breast cancer treatment.

- Support is needed from the oncology team, spouse, significant other, and family.

- Women must have the financial means to go through an adoption.

- Process of adoption may take up to several years.

❖ Nursing Issues

- Initiate discussions about the potential for amenorrhea earlier in the diagnostic and treatment phase rather than later in the survivorship experience.

✦ Discussions must occur over time and with a supportive oncology team.

✦ Amenorrhea is variable, depending on adjuvant chemotherapy dose of cyclophosphamide and patient age.

✦ There is no epidemiologic, clinical, or prognostic evidence that pregnancy or its termination will alter the natural history of breast or other cancer.

✦ Treatment has little influence on the health of offspring.

REFERENCES

1. Moore, H. (2000). Fertility and the impact of systemic therapy on hormonal status following treatment for breast cancer. *Current Oncology Reports, 2,* 587–593.

2. Koyama, H., Wada, T., Nishizawa, Y., et al. (1977). Cyclophosphamide-induced ovarian failure and its therapeutic significance in patients with breast cancer. *Cancer, 39,* 1403–1409.

3. Bines, J., Okeske, D., & Cobleigh, M. (1996). Ovarian function in premenopausal women treated with adjuvant therapy for breast cancer. *Journal of Clinical Oncology, 14,* 1718–1729.

4. Sankila, R., Heinavaara, S., & Hakulin, T. (1994). Survival of breast cancer patients after subsequent term pregnancy: "Healthy mother effect." *American Journal of Obstetrics and Gynecology, 170,* 818–823.

5. Velentgas, P., Daling, J., Malone, K., et al. (1999). Pregnancy after breast carcinoma: Outcomes and influence on mortality. *Cancer, 85,* 2424–2432, 2301–2305.

6. Blumenfeld, A., Avivi, I., Linn, S., et al. (1996). Prevention of irreversible chemotherapy-induced ovarian damage in young women with lymphoma by a gonadotrophin-releasing hormone agonist in parallel to chemotherapy. *Human Reproduction, 11,* 1620–1626.

7. Whittemore, A., Harris, R., Itnyre, J., & the Collaborative Ovarian Cancer Group. (1992). Characteristics relating to ovarian cancer risk: Collaborative analysis of 12 US case-control studies, II: Invasive epithelial ovarian cancers in white women. *American Journal of Epidemiology, 136,* 1184–1203.

8. Venn, A., Watson, L., Bruinsma, F., et al. (1999). Risk of cancer after use of fertility drugs with in-vitro fertilisation. *Lancet, 354,* 1586–1590.

9. El Hussein, E., & Tan, S. (1992). Successful in vitro fertilization and embryo transfer after treatment of invasive carcinoma of the breast. *Fertility and Sterility, 58,* 194–196.

19

Survivorship Issues

❖ Background

- ✦ *Quality of life* (QOL) is a term referring to a general sense of well-being, encompassing a multidimensional perspective including physical, psychological, social, and spiritual well-being.[1]

- ✦ Survivorship definition is based on the National Coalition for Cancer Survivorship and is defined as the process of living through and beyond a cancer diagnosis.[2]

- ✦ Breast cancer survivors include those newly diagnosed, regardless of the stage of disease; those actively receiving treatment; those having recurrence, secondary cancers, and metastatic disease; and long-term survivors without evidence of breast cancer.

- ✦ Evidence suggests that multidisciplinary models with strong clinical and advanced-practice nursing make a difference in patient satisfaction and adjustment and improve QOL.[3,4]

+ Women with breast cancer face myriad concerns after treatment ends. Many of the physical and psychological complications are described in the literature. Less evident are the social and spiritual well-being concerns.

+ Physical well-being concerns (the reader is referred to Chapters 14–18 for further discussion of these concerns)

   Lymphedema

   Menopausal symptoms

   Reproductive concerns

   Fatigue and sleep disturbance

+ Psychological well-being concerns

   Anxiety

   Depression

   Fear of recurrence and uncertainty over the future

+ Social well-being concerns

   Family relationships

+ Spiritual well-being concerns

   Meaning and purpose in life

❖ **Anxiety**[5]

   + Anxiety is a complex and universal life experience and is seen as a biobehavioral response to a stimulus that threatens one's physical, psychological, and social well-being.

+ Anxiety response involves a subjective feeling of apprehension and heightened physical arousal.

+ There are differences between anxiety as a fluctuating temporary state versus anxiety as an inherent personality trait.

+ A cognitive appraisal of the threat and stressor as potentially harmful may also produce anxiety.

+ Anxiety may influence attention, learning, and coping.

+ Risk factors for anxiety include previous mental health, older age, female gender, unrelieved physical symptoms, and concurrent medication causing anxiety.[6]

+ Assessment

> *State-Trait Anxiety Inventory (STAI) is most commonly used to measure anxiety in patients with cancer. It consists of two scales that measure the state of anxiety and the trait of anxiety.*[7]

+ In breast cancer survivors, specific points along the survivorship continuum may induce anxiety. These time points include the completion of cancer therapy; follow-up testing, procedures, and visits; change in one's oncology team; development of new breast cancer; development of recurrence and metastases; and changes in physical symptoms over time.

+ Interventions

> *Social support through groups and individual counseling*

> *Cognitive–behavioral interventions, including preparatory information, cognitive restructuring, relaxation and imagery techniques, music therapy, hypnosis, and biofeedback*

> *Educational efforts are directed at paced instruction, multiple learning opportunities through use of booklets, pamphlets, video, audio, and Internet-based information*

> *Pharmacologic management using benzodiazepines*

> *Complementary therapy* [8]

❖ **Depression** [9]

+ Depression may occur in 6% to 25% of women with breast cancer.

+ Women with advanced breast cancer have experienced higher levels of anxiety and depression (up to 25%), which may be persistent.

+ A diagnosis of breast cancer may produce mild depressive symptoms. Women with stable personalities, who have adapted well to previous life crises, usually adapt well to a diagnosis of breast cancer and are able to manage their distress.

✦ Sadness and grief are normal psychological responses for persons faced with either a threatened or an actual loss.

✦ Depressive symptoms range from mild to severe, from normal states of sadness to clinical syndromes, such as an adjustment disorder with depressed mood, or a major depression.

✦ Symptoms of depression are similar to cancer treatment effects such as fatigue, sleep pattern disturbance, changes in diet, and changes in activities of daily living.

✦ Signs and symptoms of depression

Fatigue that persists despite rest

Undifferentiated pain

Sleep disturbances in the form of insomnia or hypersomnia

Anxiety or irritability

Gastrointestinal complaints

Differentiate symptoms of disease and treatment side effects from symptoms of clinical depression.

✦ Characteristics of women at high risk

Personal or family history of depression, substance abuse, and hypochondriasis

Persistent and frequent somatic, psychosomatic, or pain complaints

History of depression before a diagnosis of breast cancer

Advanced stage of disease at diagnosis

+ Clinical evaluation[10]

Assess patient beliefs about the experience of disease and cancer treatment effects.

Diagnosis is based on clusters of symptoms that persist over time and are associated with distress and dysfunction.

+ Management of depression requires a multidisciplinary approach with appropriate individualized assessment and patient referral (Table 19-1).

❖ **Fear of Recurrence and Uncertainty over the Future**

+ Fear of recurrence, second cancers, and metastatic disease has a negative influence on psychological well-being.

+ Incidence is high and ranges from 87% to 91%.

+ Fear of recurrence may be heightened around follow-up visits and anniversary dates, and is manifested by heightened anxiety, depression, mood swings, and hypervigilance about health.

Table 19-1
Interventions for Depression

Mild depression

Validate sadness as a normal reaction to diagnosis and at various phases of the illness trajectory

Supportive understanding of the multiple personal and physical losses

Focus on grief associated with the patient's loss of health

Emphasize past strengths, support for previous effective coping strategies, and encouragement to mobilize inner resources

Assist patients in exploring and identifying their purpose in life and the role of spiritual meaning, and in determining effective coping strategies

Achieve optimal pain control and symptom management

Exercise programs and behavioral methods, such as relaxation combined with visual imagery suggesting a peaceful scene of the patient's choice

Support group referral

Moderate to severe depression

Cognitive behavioral therapy managed by clinical psychologist is aimed at controlling target symptoms

Psychotherapy interventions provided by social workers, psychiatric clinical nurse specialists, and psychologists and psychiatrists with knowledge of the specialty of oncology

Goals are to maintain a primary focus on the illness and its implications, explore issues that affect the adjustment to illness, and reinforce the patient's past coping strategies

Pharmacologic therapy may be indicated, using selective serotonin reuptake inhibitors (SSRIs)

✦ Interventions to help reduce fear of recurrence

> *Support groups have helped breast cancer survivors, within a caring environment,[11] address their fear of recurrence, metastasis, and death.*

> *One-on-one discussion and individual counseling*

> *Educating survivors with descriptive information about the need for surveillance, follow-up, and discussions about what constitutes recurrence*

> *Positive reappraisal and development of cognitive strategies to maximize coping, enhance a sense of mastery over life, and reevaluate priorities for the future*

❖ **Family Relationships[12]**

✦ Breast cancer affects the entire family, and family members have a large role in helping other family to adjust to the impact of the disease.

✦ Family members are most often identified as the primary source of emotional support for the patient.

✦ Differences between breast cancer survivors and family members

> *Perceptions of illness and degree of symptoms*

> *Subjective experiences in feelings and emotional adjustment*

> *Distress during different phases of the diagnostic, treatment, and survivorship experience*

Patterns of communication and information flow[13]

Perception of threat

+ Demands of illness

Emotional demands, with spouses reporting feelings of shock, fear, sadness, and remorse

Physical demands, with spouses taking on additional home routines, particularly during recurrence and metastatic disease

Social demands and interpersonal relationships may become strained.

Young and school-age children may have a range of reactions, including mood and self-esteem changes, academic difficulties (e.g., poor concentration and declining academic performance), somatic symptoms (e.g., stomachache, appetite changes, and difficulty sleeping), and social and interpersonal changes (e.g., acting out, withdrawal, and loss of interest).

+ Factors in helping families to adjust

Foster contact and communication with family members, who may often feel neglected.

Family-focused assessment that is not cumbersome; start with a few pointed questions about how the family is adjusting.

Direct information to both patient and family

Social support

❖ Meaning and Purpose in Life[14–16]

+ Search for meaning is a basic human need, one that is necessary for human fulfillment.

+ Deriving meaning in life is often postponed until such time that individuals face their own mortality, experience suffering, or undergo a life-changing experience, such as cancer.

+ Process of making meaning from a cancer experience may include finding a causal attribution, finding the silver lining in the experience of suffering, making downward social comparisons, searching for a higher order in the experience, and placing the cancer experience within the larger context of one's life.

+ Process of making meaning occurs over time, and the means by which one derives meaning are diverse and may include support group activities, individual counseling, keeping a journal, advocacy and activism, and volunteerism.

+ Positive outcomes of making meaning are increased coping, hopefulness, and transcendence.

+ Meaning of cancer survivorship themes were derived from the study of cancer survivors.[14]

   Having a balance between the experience of increased dependence while seeking independence and interdependence

Seeking a sense of wholeness after a life-changing experience

Facing the challenge of putting the cancer experience within the context of one's life

Struggling between elements of basic survival and reclaiming one's life

Managing physical symptoms that persist and linger over the long term

Facing multiple losses

Gaining a sense of control rather than being controlled

Contrasting the focus between seizing the day and looking to the future

+ Management

   Recognition and support for spiritual needs may fluctuate over time.

   Maintaining hope despite advancing disease

❖ Resources

+ American Cancer Society: Cancer Survivors' Network at http://cancersurvivorsnetwork.org

+ Breast Cancer Survivors Network at http://www.bcsn.org

REFERENCES

1. Dow, K. H., Ferrell, B. R., Leigh, S., et al. (1996). An evaluation of the quality of life among long-term survivors of breast cancer. *Breast Cancer Research and Treatment, 39,* 261–273.

2. Clark, E., Stovall, E., Leigh, S., et al. (1996). *Imperatives for quality cancer care: Access, advocacy, action, and accountability.* Silver Spring, MD: National Coalition for Cancer Survivorship.

3. Frost, M., Arvizu, R., Jayakumar, S., et al. (1999). A multidisciplinary healthcare delivery model for women with breast cancer: Patient satisfaction and physical and psychosocial adjustment. *Oncology Nursing Forum, 26,* 1673–1680.

4. Ritz, R., Nissen, M. J., Swenson, K., et al. (2000). Effects of advanced nursing care on quality of life and cost outcomes of women diagnosed with breast cancer. *Oncology Nursing Forum, 27,* 923–932.

5. Lehto, R., & Cimprich, B. (1999). Anxiety and directed attention in women awaiting breast cancer surgery. *Oncology Nursing Forum, 26,* 767–772.

6. Gobel, B. (2000). Anxiety. In C. H. Yarbro, M. H. Frogge, & M. Goodman (Eds.), *Cancer symptom management* (2nd ed., pp. 580–590). Sudbury, MA: Jones and Bartlett.

7. Spielberger, C., Gorush, R., & Lushene, R. (1983). *Manual for the State-Trait Anxiety Inventory.* Palo Alto, CA: Consulting Psychologists Press.

8. Stephenson, N., Weinrich, S., & Tavakoli, A. (2000). The effects of foot reflexology on anxiety and pain in patients with breast and lung cancer. *Oncology Nursing Forum, 27,* 67–72.

9. Brandt, B. (1996). Depression in women with breast cancer. In K. H. Dow (Ed.), *Contemporary issues in breast cancer* (pp. 107–120). Sudbury, MA: Jones and Bartlett.

10. McDonald, M., Passik, S., Dugan, W., et al. (1999). Nurses' recognition of depression in their patients with cancer. *Oncology Nursing Forum, 26,* 593–599.

11. Ferrell, B., Grant, M., Funk, B., et al. (1998). Quality of life in breast cancer survivors: Implications for developing support services. *Oncology Nursing Forum, 25,* 887–895.

12. Northouse, L. (1996). Spouse and family issues in breast cancer. In K. H. Dow (Ed.), *Contemporary issues in breast cancer* (pp. 163–171). Sudbury, MA: Jones and Bartlett.

13. Rees, C., & Barth, P. (2000). Exploring the information flow: Partners of women with breast cancer, patients, and healthcare professionals. *Oncology Nursing Forum, 27,* 1267–1275.

14. Dow, K. H., Ferrell, B. R., Haberman, M. R., & Eaton, L. (1999). The meaning of quality of life in cancer survivorship. *Oncology Nursing Forum, 26,* 519–528.

15. Utley, R. (1999). The evolving meaning of cancer for long-term survivors of breast cancer. *Oncology Nursing Forum, 26,* 1519–1523.

16. Taylor, E. (2000). Transformation of tragedy among women surviving breast cancer. *Oncology Nursing Forum, 27,* 781–788.

Appendix: Breast Cancer Websites

❖ **American Cancer Society**

+ http://www.cancer.org

❖ **American Society of Plastic and Reconstructive Surgeons**

+ http://www.plasticsurgery.org

❖ **American Society of Clinical Oncology**

+ http://www.asco.org

❖ **Association of Oncology Social Work**

+ http://www.biostat.wisc.edu/aosw/ aoswhello.html

❖ **Avon Breast Cancer Crusade**

+ http://www.avoncompany.com/women/ avoncrusade

❖ **BreastCancer.Net**

+ http://www.breastcancer.net

❖ **Canadian Breast Cancer Research Initiative**

  ✦ http://www.breast.cancer.ca

❖ **CancerCare Inc.**

  ✦ http://www.cancercare.org

❖ **CancerNet-Breast Cancer**

  ✦ http://cancernet.nci.nih.gov/cancer_types/
    breast_cancer.shtml

❖ **Department of Defense Breast Cancer Decision Guide**

  ✦ http://www.bcdg.org

❖ **EduCare Breast Cancer**

  ✦ http://www.cancerhelp.com/ed

❖ **Mothers Supporting Daughters with Breast Cancer**

  ✦ http://www.azstarnet.com/~pud/msdbc

❖ **National Alliance of Breast Cancer Organizations (NABCO)**

  ✦ http://www.nabco.org

❖ **National Breast Cancer Coalition**

  ✦ http://natlbcc.org

❖ **National Cancer Institute**

  ✦ http://cancernet.nci.nih.gov

❖ **National Coalition for Cancer Survivorship**

  ✦ http://www.cansearch.org

❖ **National Lymphedema Network**

  ✦ http://www.lymphnet.org

❖ **National Women's Health Information Center**

  ✦ http://www.4woman.gov

❖ **North American Menopause Society**

  ✦ http://www.menopause.org

❖ **OncoLink**

  ✦ http://cancer.med.upenn.edu/disease/breast

❖ **ONS Online**

  ✦ http://www.ons.org

❖ **Susan G. Komen Breast Cancer Foundation**

  ✦ http://www.komen.org

❖ **Y-ME National Breast Cancer Organizations**

  ✦ http://www.y-me.org

Index